rchives
of Animal Nutrition

rchiv
ür Tierernährung

OLUME 37 · JUNE 1987 · NUMBER 6

KADEMIE-VERLAG BERLIN

SSN 0003-942X Arch. Anim. Nutr.. Berlin 37 (1987) 6 467–550

Archives of Animal Nutrition covers the following topics: Biochemical and physiological foundations of animal nutrition with emphasis laid on the following aspects: Protein metabolism, metabolism of non-protein-nitrogen compounds, energy transformation, mineral metabolism, vitamin metabolism, nutritional effects and performance criteria, furthermore: practical animal feeding, feedstuff theory, feedstuff preservation and feedstuff processing.

We accept for publication:

Original manuscript not yet published in other journals and not intended for publication in other journals in the same form. Their length should not exceed 12 printed pages.

Manuscripts are to be sent to Prof. HANS BERGNER, Wissenschaftsbereich Tierernährung der Sektion Tierproduktion und Veterinärmedizin, Humboldt-Universität zu Berlin, Invalidenstr. 42, DDR - 1040 Berlin. We request the authors to submit their manuscripts typed double-spaced and ready for print. The institution which the paper originates will be mentioned together with the author's name in the title of the paper.

The author is requested to discuss and summarize the results of his work at the end of the manuscript.

Author's names in the manuscript are to be underlined with a red wavy line. We request you to underline italics with a black or blue wavy line. Small print is to be indicated by a black or blue vertical line on the margin. Bibliographic data in the text are given with the name of the author and the year of publication, in case of several publications in one year, a, b, c etc. are added according to the sequence of the publications in the bibliography, e. g. MEYER (1985a). In the bibliography the papers are arranged alphabetically according to the name of the first author and quoted as follows: surname first name, journal, volume, page and year.

Illustrations have to be restricdet to the necessary minimum and to be enclosed separately. Indicative lines, letters etc. are to be entered in pencil. For photographes, a cover sheet should be used for this. The captions of the illustrations are to be listed on an axtra sheet.

The authors receive 50 special prints of their contributions free of charge.

Terms of Subscription

Orders for the journal „Archives of Animal Nutrition" can be sent

- *in the GDR:* to the Postzeitungsvertrieb or to the Akademie-Verlag Berlin, Leipziger Str. 3–4, DDR - 1086 Berlin;
- *in the other socialist countries:* to a book-shop for foreign language literature or to the competent news-distributing agency;
- *in the FRG and Berlin (West):* to a book-shop or to the wholesale distribution agency Kunst und Wissen, Erich Bieber OHG, Wilhelmstr. 4–6, D - 7000 Stuttgart 1;
- *in the other Western European countries:* to Kunst und Wissen, Erich Bieber GmbH, General-Wille-Str. 4, Ch - 8002 Zürich;
- *in other countries:* to the international book- and journal-selling trade, to Buchexport, Volkseigener Außenhandelsbetrieb der DDR, Postfach 160, DDR - 7010 Leipzig, or to the Akademie-Verlag Berlin, Leipziger Str. 3–4, DDR - 1086 Berlin.

Zeitschrift „Archives of Animal Nutrition"

Herausgeber: Im Auftrag des Akademie-Verlages Berlin herausgegeben von Prof. Dr. Hans Bergner.

Verlag: Akademie-Verlag Berlin, Leipziger Str. 3–4, DDR - 1086 Berlin.

Fernruf: 2 23 62 01 oder 2 23 62 29, Telex-Nr.: 11 44 20.

Bank: Staatsbank der DDR Berlin Postfach 1233, Kto.-Nr.: 6836-36-20712.

Chefredakteur: Prof. Dr. sc. Hans Bergner.

Anschrift der Redaktion- Humboldt-Universität zu Berlin, Invalidenstr. 42, DDR - 1040 Berlin.

Veröffentlicht unter der Lizenznummer 1274 des Presseamtes beim Vorsitzenden
des Ministerrates der Deutschen Demokratischen Republik.

Gesamtherstellung: VEB Druckerei »Gottfried Wilhelm Leibniz«, DDR - 4450 Gräfenhainichen.

Erscheinungsweise: Archives of Animal Nutrition erscheint jährlich in einem Band mit zwölf Heften.

Bezugspreis je Band 360,– DM (zuzüglich Versandspesen); Preis je Heft 30,– DM.

Der gültige Jahresbezugspreis für die DDR ist der Postzeitungsliste zu entnehmen.

Bestellnummer dieses Heftes: 1010/37/6.

AN (EDV) 39 532

02000

ARCHIVES OF ANIMAL NUTRITION
ARCHIV FÜR TIERERNÄHRUNG
VOLUME 37 · JUNE 1987 · NUMBER 6

Arch. Anim. Nutr., Berlin 37 (1987) 6, 467–474

Forschungszentrum für Tierproduktion Dummerstorf-Rostock
Bereich Tierernährung „Oskar Kellner“
der Akademie der Landwirtschaftswissenschaften der DDR

H. PRIEBS, DORIS THOMANECK und T. HEINZ

Bestimmung der scheinbaren Verdaulichkeit des Rohproteins beim Hühnergeflügel mit Hilfe der α-NH_2-N-Methode

1. Einleitung

Die durch anatomische Besonderheiten bedingten Schwierigkeiten bei der Bestimmung der scheinbaren Verdaulichkeit des Rohproteins beim Geflügel führten zur Entwicklung verschiedener Methoden der Trennung von Kot- und Harnstickstoff. Es wurden chirurgische (Kolostomie) (GRUHN und ZIEGER, 1969) und chemische (HARTFIEL, 1963; EKMAN, 1948; TERPSTRA und DE HART, 1974) Methoden der Kot-N-Harn-N-Trennung beschrieben. Eine neue Methode der chemischen Kot-N-Harn-N-Trennung, die darauf beruht, daß der Stickstoff des Kotes und des Futters hauptsächlich als Protein gebunden bzw. als freie Aminosäure vorliegt und nach Hydrolyse kolorimetrisch mit Ninhydrin als α-NH_2-Stickstoff bestimmt werden kann, wurde von PAHLE u. a. (1983, 1985) vorgestellt. Entscheidend ist, daß der Hauptbestandteil des Harnes, die Harnsäure, bei der Hydrolyse stabil ist, und durch Ninhydrin kaum angefärbt wird.

Auf der Grundlage dieser Methode wurden von uns vergleichende Untersuchungen an Hydrolysaten von Futtermitteln und entsprechenden Mischexkrementen aus Versuchen mit kolostomierten Tieren und an Exkrementproben aus Versuchen mit intakten Tieren durchgeführt. Statt eines Aminosäureanalysators zur Bestimmung des α-NH_2-Stickstoffs wurde ein UV-VIS-Spektralphotometer verwandt. Für den Vergleich kamen auch die chemischen Methoden von HARTFIEL (1963) und EKMAN (1948) zur Anwendung. Ziel der Untersuchungen war es, das von PAHLE u. a. (1983) entwickelte Grundprinzip unter veränderten gerätetechnischen Bedingungen zu testen und bei unseren Versuchen anzuwenden.

2. Material und Methoden

Als Material für die Untersuchungen standen uns Hydrolysate von Futtermitteln, Koten, Harnen und Mischexkrementen bzw. die entsprechenden nicht hydrolysierten Proben aus Versuchen mit kolostomierten Tieren sowie Futter- und Exkrementproben aus Versuchen an intakten Tieren zur Verfügung.

Die Versuche an kolostomierten Tieren wurden im Wissenschaftsbereich Tierernährungsphysiologie und Futtermittelkunde der Sektion Tierproduktion und Veterinärmedizin der KMU Leipzig durchgeführt und uns zu Vergleichszwecken zur Verfügung gestellt. Bei der HARTFIEL-Methode wurde die Variante nach WITTENBURG und CHUDY (1967) angewandt.

Ein Teil der Untersuchungen nach HARTFIEL (1963) und EKMAN (1948) wurde parallel in verschiedenen Arbeitsgruppen durchgeführt. Den Untersuchungen zur Kot-N-Harn-N-Trennung legten wir die „Methodischen Richtlinien zur Durchführung von Verdauungsversuchen für die Futterwertschätzung" (SCHIEMANN, 1981) zugrunde.

Als Futtermittel waren in den Versuchen mit kolostomierten Tieren Gerste, Weizen und Futtermischungen (Mais/Weizen und Roggen/Weizen) und mit intakten Tieren Gerste, Gerste/Kleber, Gerste/Kleber/Strohmehl, Gerste/Kleber/Strohmehl/Stärke, Weizen/Kleber/Strohmehl, Roggen/Kleber/Strohmehl und Rapsextraktionsschrot/Fermosin eingesetzt worden.

Die Herstellung der Hydrolysate erfolgte analog der Aminosäure-Analytik. Nach einer Druckhydrolyse mit etwa 6N HCl erfolgte eine Teilneutralisation mit 40 ml Neutralisationspuffer (5 l Zitratpuffer pH 2,2 und 600 g NaOH, p. A.). Nach dem Abfiltrieren der Hydrolyserückstände wurde mit aqua dest. auf 250 ml aufgefüllt. Zur Entfernung nicht aus der Proteinfraktion stammender ninhydrinpositiver Substanzen aus den Exkrementhydrolysaten wurde jeweils 1 ml dieser Hydrolysate mit 1 ml 4 N NaOH versetzt und einer kurzen Wasserdampfdestillation unterworfen. Anschließend wurde in einen 25 ml Meßkolben überspült und aufgefüllt. Die Hydrolysate der Futtermittel wurden ohne Wasserdampfdestillation ebenfalls auf 1 : 25 verdünnt (günstiger Meßbereich für das Spektralphotometer). Die verdünnten Hydrolysate müssen sofort weiterverarbeitet werden. Von jedem Hydrolysat wurde in 3 Parallelen je 1 ml abpipettiert und mit je 1 ml Ninhydrin-Reagenz versetzt (1,6 g Ninhydrin in 60 ml 2-Methoxyethanol gelöst werden zu 20 ml 4 N Natriumazetat-Essigsäurepuffer und 100 mg $SnCl_2 \cdot 2H_2O$ gegeben. Das Ninhydrinreagenz ist täglich neu herzustellen). Anschließend wurde die gesamte Serie gleichzeitig für 20 Minuten in ein Wasserbad von 95° C gestellt. Der Abbruch der Reaktion erfolgte durch gleichzeitiges Hineinstellen der Reagenzgläser in kaltes Wasser. Anschließend wurden je 3 ml Äthanol zur Verdünnung und Farbstabilisierung hinzugegeben. Die Proben wurden nach 10 Minuten der Messung zugeführt.

Die Extinktionsmessung erfolgte mit dem UV-VIS-Spektralphotometer SPECORD M 40 (VEB Carl Zeiss Jena) gegen einen Blindwert im Vergleichsstrahlengang in 5-mm-Küvetten bei 415 und 440 nm. Der Blindwert (als Mischprobe aus 3 Einzelproben) wurde parallel zu den anderen Proben hergestellt und enthielt statt des Hydrolysats destilliertes Wasser. Gerätespezifisch wurden die Extinktionswerte der einzeln gemessenen Proben als Mittelwert von je 60 Messungen (Integrationszeit 0,5 s) ermittelt.

Von allen Proben wurden die Differenzen der Extinktionswerte E_{405}-E_{440} – ($\triangleq \Delta E$)

gebildet und auf eine einheitliche N-Einwaage (z. B. 50 mg N) umgerechnet. Der prozentuale Gehalt an Kot-Stickstoff im Exkrement ergibt sich dann aus

$$\% \text{ Kot-N} = \frac{\Delta E_{\text{Kot (50 mg)}}}{\Delta E_{\text{Futtermittel (50 mg)}}} \cdot 100$$

3. Ergebnisse und Diskussion

Das Spektrum der Reaktion ist in Abbildung 1 dargestellt und zeigt bei Messung der Farbstofflösung gegen einen Blindwert im Vergleichsstrahlengang zwei Maxima, bei 570 und 410 nm. Das veranlaßte uns, an einer großen Zahl von Proben Extinktions-

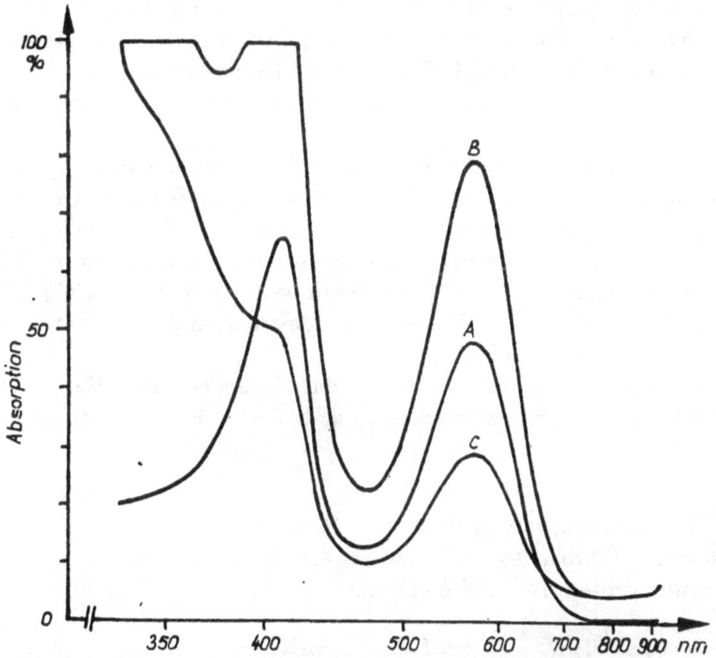

Abb. 1 (Fig. 1). Spektrum des bei der Ninhydrin-Reaktion mit Proteinhydrolysat gebildeten Farbstoffs
(Spectrum of the dye resulting from the reaction of ninhydrine with the hydrolysate of protein).
Probe gemessen gegen den Blindwert (A) und den freien Vergleichsstrahlengang (B)
C: Blindwert gemessen gegen den freien Vergleichsstrahlengang
[(Sample compared to the blank (A) and the free comparison beam (B)
C: Measurement of the blank compared to the free comparison beam)].

messungen bei verschiedenen Wellenlängen (Bereich von 415 bis 660 nm) vorzunehmen und Wellenlängendifferenzen zu bilden und zu vergleichen. Die Abweichungen waren gering, die Differenzmessung der Extinktionen bei 415 und 440 nm erwies sich am günstigsten. (Neuere Untersuchungen zeigten, daß die Messung der Extinktion nur bei 415 nm vergleichbare Werte liefert.) Die Abweichung der Meßwerte gleicher Futterproben an verschiedenen Tagen ist groß. Das hat aber keine entscheidenden Auswirkungen auf die zu bestimmende scheinbare RP-Verdaulichkeit, wenn die Ninhydrin-Reaktion mit Futter- und Exkrementhydrolysaten gleichzeitig durchgeführt wird, da dann die Relation in der Anfärberate bei beiden gleich ist. Aus diesem Grunde muß bei Wiederholungen von Messungen der Exkrementproben in jedem Fall das Futterhydrolysat als Vergleichssubstanz mitgeführt werden. Als günstig hat sich erwiesen, eine synchrone Reaktionsdurchführung mit Futter- und Exkrementhydolysaten einer Versuchsgruppe zu garantieren, um die Reaktionsbedingungen vergleichbar zu halten.

In der Literatur (zusammengefaßt u. a. bei SCHMIDT, 1965) gibt es Angaben, daß organische Lösungsmittel wie Alkohole, 1,4-Dioxan, 2-Methoxyäthanol, Pyridin und Phenole die Farbbildung beschleunigen und farbstabilisierend wirken.

Unsere Untersuchungen zur Stabilität des Farbstoffs wurden mit Humanserumalbuminhydrolysat durchgeführt. Wir konnten feststellen, daß die Farbstabilisierung in der Reihe Azeton > Propan-2-ol > Äthanol, Propan-1-ol, Butan-2-ol > Butan-1-ol > Methanol ≫ Wasser abnimmt. Bei unseren weiteren Untersuchungen nutzten wir Äthanol zur Farbstabilisierung.

Aus einem Versuch mit kolostomierten Tieren wurden die getrennt aufgefangenen Exkremente wieder vermischt und nach der α-NH_2-N-Methode untersucht. Die Ergebnisse (s. Tab. 1) zeigen, daß zwischen den nach beiden Methoden ermittelten RP-Verdaulichkeitswerten eine gute Übereinstimmung besteht. Auch zwischen den über AS-Analysator und Spektralphotometer ermittelten Werten besteht prinzipiell kein Unterschied. Die Notwendigkeit einer Wasserdampfdestillation der Exkremente (s. Tab. 1) konnte ebenfalls bestätigt werden.

Ein Methodenvergleich zwischen Kolostomie sowie den Methoden nach HARTFIEL (1963) und EKMAN (1948) mit Mischexkrementen aus Kolostomieversuchen zeigte

Tabelle 1 (Table 1)

Methodenvergleich zur Bestimmung der scheinbaren Rohproteinverdaulichkeit in % (2 Methoden) (Comparison of methods for determination of the digestibility of crude protein in %, 2 methods)

Tier-Nr. (No. of animal)	Kolostomie (Colostomy)	α-NH_2-N (α-amino-N) (AAA)	α-NH_2-N (α-amino-N) (SPECORD)	α-NH_2N* (α-amino-N) (SPECORD)
1	76,5	77,8	79,2	63,8
2	77,7	78,3	78,6	67,9
3	79,8	80,0	78,8	65,4
4	80,2	78,9	77,8	63,3
5	79,0	79,6	77,4	66,0
$\bar{x}$, s	78,6 ± 1,5	78,9 ± 0,9	78,4 ± 0,7	65,3 ± 1,8

α-NH_2-N (AAA) (α-amino-N) – mit Hilfe des modifizierten Aminosäureanalysators erhaltene Werte (Measured values using an modified amino acid analyzer)

α-NH_2-N (SPECORD) (α-amino-N) – mit Hilfe des UV-VIS Spektralphotometers SPECORD M 40 erhaltene Werte nach Wasserdampfdestillation (Measured values after water steam distillation using the UV-VIS-Spectrophotometer SPECORD M 40)

α-NH_2-N* (SPECORD) (α-amino-N) – ohne Wasserdampfdestillation (Without water steamdistillation)

Tabelle 2 (Table 2)

Methodenvergleich zur Bestimmung der scheinbaren Rohproteinverdaulichkeit in % verschiedener Futtermittel (4 Methoden) (Comparison of methods for determination of the apparent digestibility of crude protein in % of different feeds, 4 methods)

Futtermittel (Feeds)	n*	Methode (Method)			
		Kolostomie (Colostomy) $\bar{x} \pm s$	HARTFIEL $\bar{x} \pm s$	EKMAN $\bar{x} \pm s$	α-NH_2-N (α-amino-N) $\bar{x} \pm s$
Weizen 1 (Wheat 1)	6	82,6 ± 6,3	70,6 ± 5,3	75,3 ± 9,8	81,5 ± 6,0
Weizen 2 (Wheat 2)	4	80,9 ± 1,1	n. b.	89,7 ± 3,1	77,9 ± 3,6
Gerste 1 (Barley 1)	4	73,5 ± 5,2	68,3 ± 4,8	75,2 ± 7,0	73,4 ± 4,5
Gerste 2 (Barley 2)	3	69,5 ± 9,3	n. b.	83,3 ± 5,8	69,0 ± 13,3
Mais/Weizen (Corn/wheat)	3	83,5 ± 1,1	84,7 ± 1,4	89,4 ± 1,6	79,6 ± 2,6
Roggen/Weizen (Rye/wheat)	3	81,9 ± 0,7	73,9 ± 2,2	84,6 ± 0,1	71,3 ± 1,7

n. b. = nicht bestimmt (Not determined)
* = Anzahl der Exkrementproben (Number of excrement samples)

Tabelle 3 (Table 3)

Methodenvergleich zur Bestimmung des Gehaltes an Kot-N (in % vom Gesamtexkrement-N) in Hühnerexkrementen (Comparison of methods for determination of the content of the faecal-N in % related to the total amount of the excrement-N of chicken)

Tier-Nr. (No. of animal)	Kolostomie (Colostomy)	Methoden (Methods) α-NH_2-N (α-amino-N)	H_1	H_2	E_1	E_2
1	28,8	29,7	33,4	33,9	29,0	39,1
2	21,9	23,0	30,5	42,7	16,2	37,6
3	18,4	20,9	31,1	42,3	15,3	27,7
4	21,1	24,9	40,8	40,5	22,8	26,3
5	20,6	20,7	21,7	36,0	17,5	38,6
6	25,6	27,2	35,7	40,7	19,1	42,8
7	36,8	36,5	40,7	48,5	29,3	32,0
8	42,7	45,8	45,9	49,2	22,5	36,1
9	43,1	40,5	54,9	48,5	27,8	40,7
10	29,3	32,3	28,8	36,5	22,0	52,0
$\bar{x}_{1-6}$	22,7	24,4	32,2	39,4	20,0	35,4
$\bar{x}_{7-10}$	38,0	38,8	42,6	45,7	25,4	40,2

H_1, H_2, E_1, E_2 – unterschiedliche Arbeitsgruppen bei den Methoden nach HARTFIEL bzw. EKMAN (Different working groups for methods by HARTFIEL and EKMAN resp.)
(Die Tiere 1–6 erhielten Weizen, die Tier 7–10 Gerste)
(Feeding of animals 1–6 with wheat and 7–10 with barley, resp.)

ebenfalls eine gute Übereinstimmung zwischen Kolostomie und α-NH_2-N-Methode (SPECORD M 40) bei Weizen und Gerste als Alleinfuttermittel (Tab. 2).

Dagegen zeigen die Ergebnisse nach der HARTFIEL-Methode bzw. EKMAN-Methode z. T. beträchtliche Differenzen zur Kolostomie. Nach der EKMAN-Methode wurden in der Regel etwas höhere scheinbare RP-Verdaulichkeiten ermittelt, wogegen die der HARTFIEL-Methode fast ausschließlich niedriger waren. Abweichungen gab es auch zwischen Kolostomie und modifizierter α-NH_2-N-Methode bei den angeführten Futtermischungen, für die keine Erklärung gegeben werden kann.

Zur Klärung der Differenzen in den Methoden nach HARTFIEL (1963) und EKMAN (1948) wurden Untersuchungen an Mischexkrementen aus Versuchen mit Weizen 1 und Gerste 1 (s. Tab. 2) durch verschiedene Arbeitsgruppen durchgeführt und mit den Ergebnissen der Kolostomie und der modifizierten α-NH_2-N-Methode verglichen (Tab. 3). Um die methodischen Unzulänglichkeiten der HARTFIEL- und EKMAN-Methode sichtbar zu machen, sind hier die Mittelwerte des Kot-N-Gehaltes (%) für jedes Versuchstier nach allen genannten Methoden angegeben. Aus diesen Beispielen geht wiederum eine gute Übereinstimmung der Mittelwerte je Tier zwischen der Kolostomie und der modifizierten α-NH_2-N-Methode hervor. Sowohl bei der HARTFIEL- als auch bei der EKMAN-Methode traten bis auf wenige Ausnahmen große Abweichungen zum entsprechenden Kolostomie-Wert auf. Auch zwischen den verschiedenen Arbeitsgruppen gibt es bis auf wenige Werte keine Übereinstimmung. Das spricht eindeutig für eine schlechtere Handhabbarkeit dieser Methoden.

Wegen der besseren Übereinstimmung der Werte aus der Kolostomie und der α-NH_2-N-Methode entschlossen wir uns, eine Reihe von Untersuchungen zum Vergleich

Tabelle 4 (Table 4)

Methodenvergleich zur Bestimmung der scheinbaren Rohprotein-Verdaulichkeit in %
(Exkremente von intakten Tieren)
(Comparison of methods for determination of apparent digestibility of crude protein in %, excrements of non operated chicken)

Futtermittel (Feeds)	n	α-NH_2-N (α-amino-N)	Methoden (Methods) HARTFIEL	EKMAN
Gerste (Barley)	5	71,5 ± 2,7	72,0 ± 2,0	86,4 ± 7,6
Gerste/Weizenkleber (Barley/wheat gluten)	5	85,7 ± 3,2	91,3 ± 3,2	101,6 ± 9,0
Gerste/Weizenkleber/Strohmehl (Barley/wheat gluten/straw meal)	5	75,5 ± 3,9	87,8 ± 4,1	97,4 ± 9,9
Gerste/Weizenkleber/Strohmehl/Stärke (Barley/wheat gluten/straw meal/starch)	5	78,2 ± 5,4	74,6 ± 5,7	85,0 ± 3,6
Weizen/Weizenkleber/Strohmehl (Wheat/wheat gluten/straw meal)	7	84,7 ± 1,5	n. b.	74,2 ± 9,2
Roggen/Weizenkleber/Strohmehl (Rye/wheat gluten/straw meal)	8	78,1 ± 1,7	n. b.	73,4 ± 5,6
RES/Fermosin* (Rapeseed meal/Fermosin)*	6	84,3 ± 2,0	84,1 ± 1,4	84,9 ± 3,8

* Fermosin – Hefe aus Erdöldestillaten (Yeast from oil distillates)
RES – Rapsextraktionsschrot (Rapeseed solvent-extracted meal)

dieser Methoden mit denen nach HARTFIEL (1963) und EKMAN (1948) durchzuführen. Dazu wurden die Exkrementproben aus Versuchen an intakten Tieren (Zuchthähne) herangezogen und die scheinbare RP-Verdaulichkeit der eingesetzten Futtermittel nach den verschiedenen Methoden ermittelt (Tabelle 4). Wie schon in den Untersuchungen mit Mischexkrementen aus Versuchen mit kolostomierten Tieren zeigte sich auch hier eine ungenügende Übereinstimmung der Ergebnisse von HARTFIEL- und EKMAN-Methode mit denen der α-NH_2-N-Methode (Ausnahme: RES/Fermosin-Futterhefe). Auffallend ist, daß nach der EKMAN-Methode zum Teil irreale Werte für die scheinbare RP-Verdaulichkeit ermittelt wurden, bei denen die Standardabweichung um ein Vielfaches höher war als in den gleichen Versuchen nach der α-NH_2-N- bzw. HARTFIEL-Methode.

Die hier vorgestellten Ergebnisse sprechen für die Eignung der modifizierten α-NH_2-N-Methode nach PAHLE u. a. (1983, 1985) zur Kot-N-Harn-N-Trennung. Diese Methode erweist sich auch als günstig wegen eines erheblich höheren Probendurchlaufs.

Zusammenfassung

Auf der Grundlage eines Vergleichs zwischen der Kolostomie, der von PAHLE u. a. (1983, 1985) vorgestellten α-NH_2-N-Methode und der Methoden nach HARTFIEL (1963) sowie EKMAN (1948) zur Kot-N-Harn-N-Trennung bei der Bestimmung der scheinbaren Verdaulichkeit des Rohproteins am Hühnergeflügel wurden umfangreiche Untersuchungen mit Mischexkrementen aus Kolostomie-Versuchen und Exkrementproben von intakten Tieren aus Verdaulichkeitsversuchen mit unterschiedlichen Futtermitteln durchgeführt. Bei der Anwendung der Methoden von HARTFIEL und EKMAN wurden z. T. große Abweichungen in den Meßergebissen festgestellt. Eine von uns angewandte Modifizierung der α-NH_2-N-Methode führte zu Ergebnissen, die in guter Übereinstimmung mit den Ergebnissen der Kolostomie und der von PAHLE entwickelten Methode standen.

Резюме

Х. Прибс, Дорис Томанек и Т. Хайнц

Опеределение видимой переваримости сырого протеина с помощью α-NH_2-N у птиц

На основе сравнения между способом колостомирования, методом α-NH_2-N Пале и др. (1983, 1985) и способом Хартфила (1963) и Экмана (1948) для деления азота в кале и в моче при определении видимой переваримости сырого протеина у птиц проводились многочисленные исследования, где взялись смешанные экскременты из колостомированных опытов и тоже пробы от неоперированных птиц из переваримых опытов с применением различных кормов. При применении методов Хартфила и Экмана обнаружили значительные отклонения полученных данных. Применяемой нами модифицированный способ α-NH_2-N вёл к результатам, которые хорошо совпадали с результатами, полученными при колостомизации или с помощью метода Пале.

Summary

H. PRIEBS, DORIS THOMANECK and T. HEINZ

Determination of the apparent digestibility of crude protein in chickens by means of the α-NH_2-N- method

Based on a comparison between colostomy, the α-NH_2-N method introduced by PAHLE et al. (1983, 1985), the HARTFIEL (1963) and the EKMAN (1948) methods of the separation of faecal N and urine N in the determination of the apparent digestibility of crude protein in chickens, extensive studies were carried out with mixed excrement from colostomy experiments and excrement samples from intact animals from digestibility experiments with different feedstuffs. In case of the application of the methods by HARTFIEL and EKMAN there were partly big deviations in the measured results. A modification of the α-NH_2-N method applied by us showed results wich largely agreed with the results of colostomy and the method developed by PAHLE.

Literaturverzeichnis

[1] EKMAN, P.: Eighth World's Poultry Congress, Copenhagen **1**, 222 (1948)
[2] GRUHN, K. und M. ZIEGER: Arch. Tierernähr. **19**, 631 (1969)
[3] HARTFIEL, W.: Chemische Untersuchungen bei Stoffwechselversuchen mit Hühnern. Diss., Verlag Bonn (1963)
[4] PAHLE, T., ROSEMARIE KÖHLER, INGRID HALLE, H. JEROCH und G. GEBHARDT: Arch. Tierernähr. **33**, 363 (1983)
[5] PAHLE, T., ROSEMARIE KÖHLER, INGRID HALLE, H. JEROCH und G. GEBHARDT: Arch. Tierernähr. **35**, 81 (1985)
[6] SCHIEMANN, R.: Arch. Tierernähr. **31**, 1 (1981)
[7] SCHMICT, R.-D.: Beiträge zur säulenchromatographischen Analytik der essentiellen Aminosäuren Cystin/Cystein, Methionin, Lysin und zum Reaktionsablauf der Ninhydrin-Aminosäure-Farbreaktion. Diss. (Prom. A), Quedlinburg (1965)
[8] TERPSTRA, K. und N. DE HART: Z. Tierphysiol. Tierernähr. Futtermittelkde. **32**, 306 (1974)
[9] WITTENBURG, H. und A. CHUDY: Arch. Geflügelzucht und Kleintierk. **16**, 221 (1967)

Unser Dank gilt Herrn Dr. PAHLE für die Hinweise und die Bereitstellung von Proben kolostomierter Tiere, sowie den Mitarbeiterinnen Frau URSULA POHLMANN, Frau EDELTRAUT JENSSEN und Frau BÄRBEL ENGLER für die Durchführung der Verdaulichkeitsversuche und die Bearbeitung der Proben.

Eingegangen: 9. Dezember 1985

Anschriften der Autoren:

Dr. H. PRIEBS
Forschungszentrum für Tierproduktion Dummerstorf-Rostock,
Bereich WO,
Dummerstorf
DDR - 2551

DORIS THOMANECK und Dr. THOMAS HEINZ:
Forschungszentrum für Tierproduktion Dummerstorf-Rostock,
Bereich Tierernährung „Oskar Kellner“
Justus-von-Liebig-Str. 2, Fach-Nr. 27-02
Rostock
DDR - 2500

Arch. Anim. Nutr., Berlin 37 (1987) 6, 475–488

National Institute for Research in Dairying, Shinfield, Reading, RG2 9AT, England

R. J. Merry, R. H. Smith and A. B. McAllan

Studies of rumen function in an *in vitro* continuous culture system

1. Introduction

Because of the difficulties encountered in *in vivo* studies, a number of *in vitro* techniques aimed at simulating some aspects of rumen function, have been developed. These range from simple batch culture systems to more complex continuous culture methods which were reviewed by Ewart (1974) and Czerkawski (1976, 1986). More recently, studies of this kind have been reported by Crawford et al., 1980 a, b; Stern, 1984 and Abe & Kurihara (1984). The main attraction of an *in vitro* system is the degree of control and convenience it affords.

Simple batch culture systems have been used to obtain basic information regarding degradative and synthetic processes in the rumen, but the analogy of the rumen with continuous culture has long been recognised (Hobson, 1965). A number of systems using continuous or semi-continuous techniques have been developed; a successful and widely used method is that of Czerkawski & Breckenridge (1977). In this system feed is physically restrained in polyester bags within the vessel and changed periodically. Another approach is that of Hoover et al. (1976a) in which solid feed is added continuously to a fermenter and both solid and liquid outflow rates are controlled.

The apparatus described in the present paper is based upon that of Hoover et al. (1976 a). Its special features and some experiments defining the processes it supports are described. Some of this work has been published briefly elsewhere (Merry et al., 1984 a, b).

2. Materials and Methods

2.1. Donor animals and collection of digesta

Three Suffolk wethers (60–70 kg), each equipped with a cannula in the dorsal sac of the rumen were used as donor animals for rumen contents to charge the continuous culture vessels. They were given a daily diet (kg/d) of chopped barley straw (0.45 kg), rolled barley (0.45 kg), white fishmeal (0.10 kg) and urea (0.01 kg). The diet was given in two equal amounts at 09.00 and 16.00 h. This diet was broadly similar to those used in subsequent *in vitro* experiments.

2.2. Equipment

The complete continuous culture system is shown diagramatically in Fig. 1. The automatic feeder consisted of a PVC tube (A) with a piston (B) operated by a variable speed drive motor. The piston pushed a stainless steel rod (C) with detachable plastic

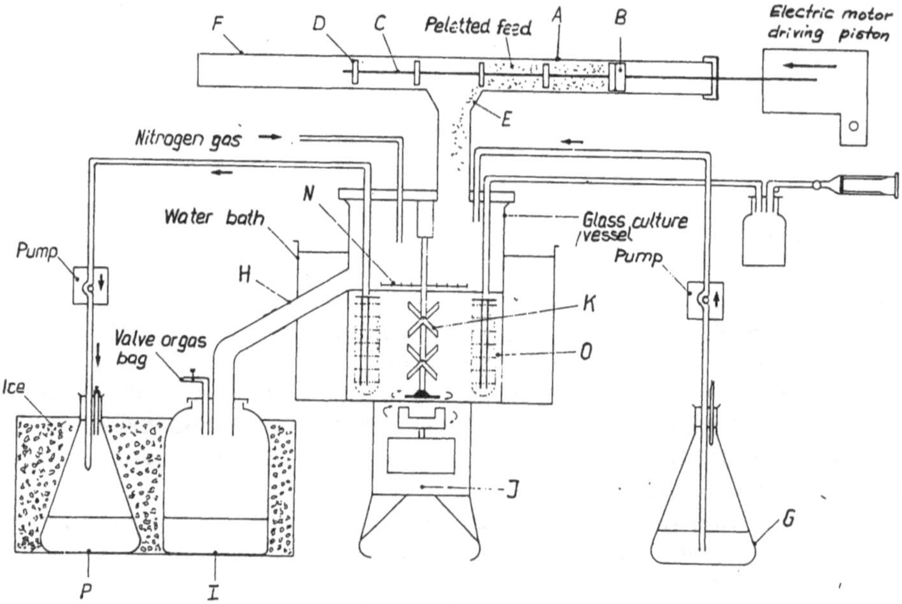

Fig. 1. Continuous culture apparatus: A. PVC tube; B. piston; C. stainless steel rod; D. plastic spacer; E. T-piece funnel; F. extension tube; G. artificial saliva reservoir; H. sidearm; I. displaced effluent collection vessel; J. magnetic stirrer; K. impeller; O. filter; P. filtered effluent collection vessel.

spacers (D) between which pelleted feed was packed. In this way compaction of the pellets was avoided and feed entered the fermenter vessel, via a T-piece funnel (E), virtually continuously. Rod C passed into the extension tube F. The feeder was initially charged with pelleted feed sufficient for 24 h and replenished at the end of each 24 h period by exchanging the empty tube for a full one. Artificial saliva (G) (McDOUGALL, 1948, diluted 60 : 40 with distilled water) adjusted to pH 9.0 by adding NaOH, and containing 0.025 % (w/v) cysteine monohydrochloride was pumped continuously into the vessel as shown (Fig. 1).

The fermenter vessel (Fig. 2) was of glass (Primarc Jigs & Lamps, Reading, Berkshire) and was initially charged with strained rumen contents from the donor sheep and immersed in a water bath at 39 °C. The vessel was fitted with a side-arm (22 mm I. D.) (H) at a height allowing a liquid volume of 1180 ml within the vessel before overflow. Effluent which overflowed (displaced effluent) passed into a cooled collection vessel (I) (Fig. 1). The rim of the culture vessel was flared to a diameter of 150 mm and ground. The lid, fitted with a butyl rubber seal was held in position with clamps. The lid had a large port (28 mm diameter) for feed entry and smaller ports (12 mm diameter) for infusion or sampling purposes (see Fig. 2 for lay-out). A magnetic stirrer (LH Engi-

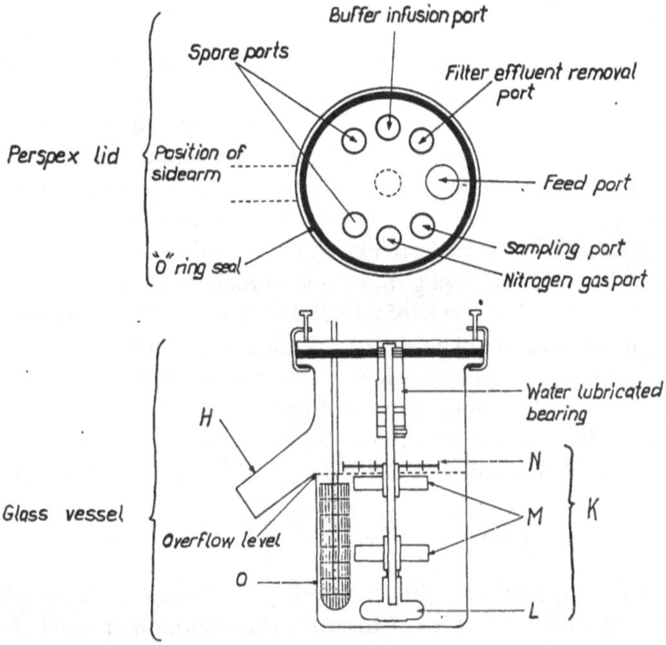

Fig. 2. Continuous culture vessel and impeller system, and lid showing positions of entry and exit ports. H. sidearm; K. impeller; L. bar magnet; M. mixing paddles; N. foam breaker; O. filter.

neering, Stoke Poges, Bucks) (J) (Fig. 1) was situated beneath the culture vessel and controlled by a timing device which allowed either continuous or intermittent mixing. The stirrer drove an impeller (K) with a bar magnet (L) (LH Engineering, Stoke Poges, Bucks), which had two sets of mixing paddles (M) and a foam breaker (N) (Fig. 2). Nitrogen gas was introduced continuously into the head space of the vessel. Two filters (0) were immersed in the vessel contents with tubes leading through two of the smaller entry ports in the lid (Fig. 2). Each consisted of a stainless steel mesh former covered by a polyester sac (200 µm pore size). Filtered effluent containing little solid material, was pumped continuously through one filter and entered a cooled collection vessel (P) (Fig. 1). Daily samples of vessel contents were removed through the other filter using a syringe, before replenishing the feed supply. The collection vessels were sealed, except for Bunsen valves permitting the discharge of fermentation gases. It would have been possible to collect these gases if required but in the present experiments they were simply vented to the atmosphere. Contents of both collection vessels (I & P) were removed at 24 h intervals at the same time that the feed tube was replenished.

2.3. Inoculum source

On the first day of an experiment samples of rumen contents (approximately 1.5 l) were taken from each of the 3 donor sheep before a morning feed, by suction through a perforated tube (ID. 20 mm). The 3 samples of rumen contents were pooled, strained through 4 layers of surgical gauze, and used to charge the culture vessels within approximately 15 min of collection.

2.4. Solid feed and infusates entering the vessel

A diet was prepared from (g/kg) barley (270), barley straw (480), tapioca (80), fishmeal (150) and urea (10). The straw was ground to pass through a 4 mm screen and the barley and tapioca were ground to pass through a 2 mm screen. The barley, straw, fishmeal and tapioca were mixed thoroughly with water (1.3 l/kg diet) containing methyl cellulose (10 g/kg) and the urea for 3 h, and then pelleted. The pellets were dried at 30 ° for 48 h and reduced in size to approximately 5 mm lengths. Using values from published information (ARC, 1980; MAFF, 1975) it was calculated that the diet contained 14.8 g rumen degradable N (RDN)/kg DM and 449 g digestible organic matter/kg DM.

The dietary pellets were introduced at a rate of 33 g DM/day and artificial saliva was infused continuously at approximately 79 ml/h by the peristaltic pump during the period (up to 19 d) that an experiment continued. Withdrawal rate of filtered effluent was set at 32 ml/h. During periods where microbial growth was being monitored, 100 μCi (0.05 μCi/ml) $NaH_2{}^{32}PO_4$ (Amersham International, Amersham) were included in the artifical saliva and infused continuously for at least 8 d before sampling began.

2.5. Sampling procedure and preparation of samples

During an experiment, samples of filtered effluent and displaced effluent were taken daily just after replenishing the feed. Samples of filtered effluent and displaced effluent were combined in proportion to the amounts collected (mixed effluent). Where appropriate a small sample of mixed effluent (25 g) was extracted as described in section 2.6 for determination of ^{32}P activity. Other samples of mixed effluent, filtered effluent and displaced effluent (200 g) were frozen at −20 °C for subsequent analyses of volatile fatty acids, dry matter, ammonia and carbohydrates.

Bacteria were harvested from a one litre sample of mixed effluent on day 12 and sometimes day 19 and from total vessel contents at the end of the experiment, according to the procedure of SMITH & MCALLAN (1974). Part of each sample of separated bacteria was extracted as described in section 2.6 for subsequent ^{32}P counting, and the remainder deep-frozen (−20 °C) to await analysis of N, dry matter and carbohydrates.

Daily samples (10 ml) were taken of filtered vessel contents and pH and redox potential measured immediately. To 2 ml of the sample was added 0.05 ml of 0.1 % (w/v) formalin in 10 % (w/v) sodium chloride solution and the mixture retained for counting protozoa. Hydrochloric acid (0.6 ml; 2 M) was added to another 3 ml of the sample with mixing, the mixture centrifuged (10 min. at 35000 g) and the supernatant frozen for subsequent analysis of ammonia. The rest of the sample was centrifuged at 35000 g for 10 min. and the supernatants retained for inorganic-P analysis and ^{32}P counting.

2.6. Measurement of microbial-N flow

Samples of mixed effluent obtained during periods of ^{32}P infusion were extracted immediately after collection with acid and lipid solvents as described by MCALLAN & SMITH (1969), to prepare a residue from which all the P had been removed except that bound in the form of nucleic acid. This sample was digested, and counted on a liquid scintillation counter as described by MERRY et al. (1982), to give a measure of ^{32}P–

laelled nucleic acid. At the same time nucleic acid-P and total N were determined in corresponding samples of harvested, mixed rumen bacteria. Microbial N in the mixed effluent sample was estimated as

$$\frac{^{32}\text{P mixed effluent}}{^{32}\text{P/N bacteria}}$$

2.7. Analytical methods

Ammonia-N and protozoal numbers were determined according to MERRY (1980) and total and urea-N were determined by the methods of SMITH & McALLAN (1970) and MERRY et al. (1982) respectively.

Inorganic-P, DM and OM were determined as described by SMITH et al. (1978) and carbohydrates by the method of McALLAN & SMITH (1974). Volatile fatty acids were determined in supernatants of mixed effluent as described by MERRY (1980).

2.8. Statistical treatment

Variation between experiments (Se^2) and variation between days of sampling within experiments (Sd^2) were calculated. These values were used to derive variance components for experiments (δ_e^2) and days (δ_d^2). From these values were calculated sets of means of combinations of different numbers of experiments and days of sampling using the equation shown below.

$$\sqrt{\frac{n_d \cdot \delta_e^2 + \delta_d^2}{n_e \cdot n_d}}$$

The results were expressed as percentages of each overall mean.

3. Results

3.1. Establishing a steady state

Of the four replicate experiments, (each with a fresh inoculum) carried out over 12-day periods, two were continued for another 7 days to study further the time needed for a steady-state to be established and its stability assessed.

The values shown in Fig. 3 indicated that the dry matter content of filtered effluent decreased and that for displaced effluent increased in the first few days but that after 5 days both values reached a plateau (approximately 1.3 and 2.5 % respectively). Changes with time in other characteristics of the system are illustrated in Fig. 4. A reasonably constant pH value of approximately 6.7 was achieved by 5 days and after that time redox potential was always more negative than -300 mV. Protozoal numbers declined in the first few days of an experiment but then stabilized to give counts of approximately 3×10^4 (principally *Entodinia* spp.) as long as the experiment continued. Total volatile fatty acid (TVFA) concentration increased and ammonia concentration decreased sharply during the initial period of the experiment but both then remained reasonably conssant.

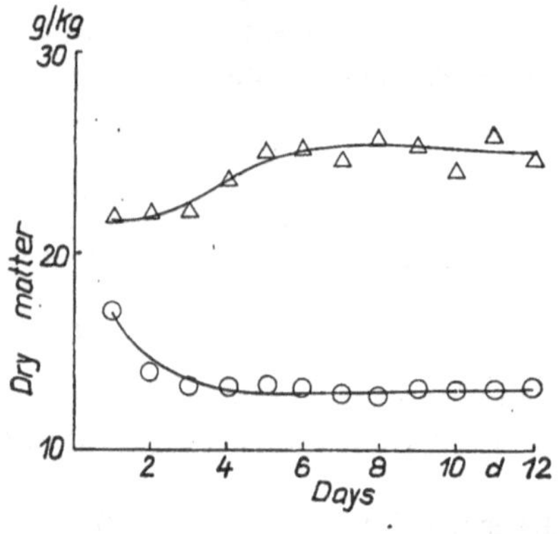

Fig. 3. Dry matter content of filtered (○) and displaced (△) effluent from continuous cultures of mixed rumen contents. Results are mean values for 2 experiments.

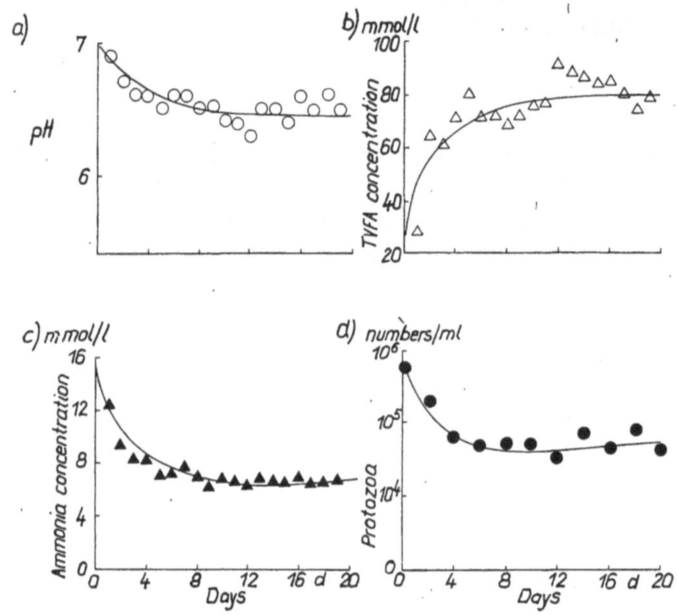

Fig. 4. Daily values for a. vessel pH (○); b. effluent total volatile fatty acid (TVFA) concentration (△); c. vessel ammonia concentration (▲) and d. vessel protozoal numbers (●) in continuous culture of rumen contents. Results for days 1–12 are mean values for 4 replicate experiments and days 13–19 for 2 replicate experiments. Cultures were fed a diet of barley, straw and tapioca supplemented with fishmeal and urea (see p. 478). Effluent samples were prepared as described on p. 478.

All these observations indicate that a steady-state in the model rumen can be assumed after 5 days and the comparisons in Table 1 showing little difference between pooled samples for days 8–12 on the one hand and days 15–19 on the other, confirm this view.

Table 1

Effect of time of incubation on some measurements made on vessel contents or effluents from a continuous culture of rumen contents

	Days 8–12 mean	*S. E.*	Days 15–19 mean	*S. E.*
Vessel pH	6.75	0.053	6.67	0.047
Vessel ammonia concentration (m mol/l)	12.1	0.75	13.4	0.79
Effluent total volatile fatty acid:				
Concentration (m mol/l)	86.2	2.66	84.0	2.78
Flow (m mol/d)	143.0	3.09	137.4	3.77
Microbial N flow (g/d)	0.49	0.023	0.52	0.040

Results are means values for 2 experiments in which samples were taken daily during the periods shown (i.e. $n = 10$). Continuous cultures were fed diets supplemented with fishmeal and urea.

3.2. Estimating the extent of microbial synthesis

Fig. 5 shows the changes in specific activity in the inorganic P in samples from the model rumen after starting to include $Na^{32}PO_4$ in the artificial saliva from day 4. It also shows changes in synthesized microbial N flow estimated in the manner described on p. 478 These estimates depended upon obtaining a reliable value for ^{32}P : N ratio in

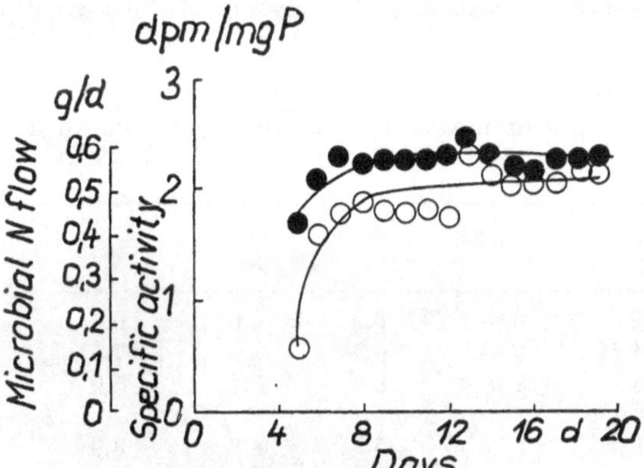

Fig. 5. Changes in specific activity of inorganic P pool (●; dpm/mg P) and microbial N flow (○; g/d) in continuous cultures of rumen contents. Results are mean values for 4 experiments up to and including day 12 and for 2 experiments from day 13 to day 19, ^{32}P infusion commenced on day 4 and cultures were fed a diet of barley, straw and tapioca supplemented with fishmeal and urea (see p. 478).

the bacteria in the vessel. In four comparisons mean values (dpm $\times 10^{-3}$/mg N) with standard errors for bacterial samples separated from mixed effluent (collected in ice during 24 h), and from total vessel content (extracted immediately after collection) were 25.8 (1.8) and 25.4 (2.2) respectively. The fact that these values were closely similar indicated that it is satisfactory to employ effluent samples collected in ice for 24 h for this purpose.

It was apparent that a steady-state in the labelling of the inorganic P pool was achieved in less than 2 days and that estimates of microbial N flow were nearly constant from that time (Fig. 5). The latter finding was indicated also by the results given in Table 1; as was found for the other rumen characteristics there was little difference between estimates of microbial N flow made on pooled samples for days 8–12 and days 15–19 respectively.

3.3. Characteristics of the system at steady-state

As discussed above, the values in Table 1 were shown after a steady-state had been achieved. Under these conditions (i.e. at least 5 days after starting the experiment) with an artificial saliva input rate of 79 ml/h, the mean (SE) values (kg/d) for filtered and displaced effluent flows in the 4 experiments were 0.75 (0.004) and 0.91 (0.006) respectively. This corresponded to a fractional liquid turnover rate of 0.064/h and an organic matter (OM) turnover rate of 0.034/h. The difference between these rates reflected mainly the exclusion of large particle OM from the filtered effluent and indicated a mean retention time of approximately 30 h for these particles.

Although the filtered effluent was not completely free of particulate matter, mean (SE) estimates of flows of bound carbohydrates at steady-state (based on pooled 8–12 day samples) in filtered effluent as proportions of total outflows, were only 0.06 (0.02), 0.02 (0.01), 0.07 (0.02) and 0.16 (0.01) for arabinose, xylose, β-linked ('cellulose') glucose and α-linked ('starch') glucose respectively.

3.4. Variability of measurements

In order to predict possible variations in measurements with experimental conditions other than those reported in this paper, standard erros of means were calculated for combinations of days of sampling (range 1–10) and numbers of replicate experiments (range 2–8). Selected values are presented in Table 2. In the present studies where 4

Table 2

Predicted variation (%) in standard errors of means for measurements made in a continuous culture system

Number of experiments		2			4	
Number of days	1	3	5	1	3	5
pH	1.4	0.9	0.8	0.9	0.6	0.5
Ammonia	13.1	11.1	10.6	9.3	7.9	7.5
Total volatile fatty acid	7.4	7.1	7.0	5.2	5.1	5.0
Microbial N	7.5	5.9	5.7	5.3	4.3	3.9
Arabinose	11.8	7.0	5.5	8.2	4.8	3.9
Xylose	12.8	8.1	6.9	9.0	5.8	4.9
β-linked ('cellulose') glucose	14.1	11.6	11.0	10.0	8.2	7.8

Values were calculated as described on p. 479 and are expressed as percentages of each overall mean obtained in 4 experiments with 5 days of sampling.

replicate experiments were performed with 5 days of sampling, variation from the overall mean was less than 5 % for the majority of measurements made. Slightly greater variation for β-linked ('cellulose') glucose has subsequently been overcome by freeze-drying samples, to concentrate them before analysis (R. J. MERRY, unpublished observations). Values presented in Table 2 suggest that increasing the number of experiments would lead to greater reduction in variation than increasing the number of sampling days. For example, where 6–8 experiments were carried out with 5 days of sampling, variation could be reduced to less than 4 %.

4. Discussion

The main difficulties associated with simulating the rumen *in vitro*, are: (i) maintaining, in the presence of a solid substrate, a balanced microbial population which is fairly representative of that present in the rumens of animals fed the diet under test, and (ii) simply and accurately manipulating flows of particulate digesta out of the vessel. For studies of factors affecting microbial growth and fibre digestion these are both prime requirements. A system similar to that described has been used by a number of workers (HOOVER et al., 1976 a, b; CRAWFORD et al., 1980 a, b; STERN et al., 1978) to study rumen digestion, in experiments lasting fairly short periods (usually no longer than 8 days). The present work included an evaluation for a longer period.

In preliminary experiments it was found that several modifications were necessary to meet our experimental requirements. In the system developed by HOOVER et al. (1976 a, b) cultures were fed semi-continuously over 4×3-hourly periods with alternate spells of 3 h where no feed entered the vessel. We considered this method of feeding unsatisfactory as it would lead to fluctuation in conditions within the vessel. To improve upon this we introduced a system of thin spacers, mounted on stainless steel rods inside the feed tubes, between which pelleted feed was packed. This prevented compaction in the tubes and allowed a virtually continuous input of feed. Other modifications were a reduction in vessel size for convenience, and provision of a foam breaker (a stainless steel rod with cross-pieces which moved across the surface of the vessel contents). In addition the system was completely sealed, except for an outlet where gases could either be vented to the atmosphere via a non-return valve or could be collected if complete input/output balances were to be made. We also abandoned any attempt to completely remove suspended matter from the filtered effluent. The use of very fine mesh cloth as proposed by HOOVER et al. (1976 a) caused severe difficulties with blockage when the system was run for more than a short period. As the main objective of manipulating relative flows of solid and liquid digesta could be achieved with only partial removal of solid particles, we routinely employed filter cloth with a larger pore size (200 μm), which did not block, but greatly reduced the DM content of filtered effluent compared to displaced effluent.

One factor commonly thought to be important in *in vitro* continuous culture models of the rumen is the extent of protozoal survival. Some early systems only maintained protozoa for very short periods (RUFENER et al., 1963; SLYTER at al., 1964; DAVEY et al., 1966). More recently there has been greater success (HOOVER et al., 1976 a, b; CZERKAWSKI & BRECKENRIDGE, 1977) in systems where large solid particles can be retained in the vessel for extended periods. Under the conditions used in the present experiments total numbers declined in the first 4 days to $3–5 \times 10^4$/ml, which represented a 10-fold reduction in numbers compared to the original inoculum. The principal types found after this time were small *Entodinia* spp. but numbers remained constant for up to 21 d. An initial fall in protozoal numbers was also observed by HOOVER *et al.* (1976 b). In vivo, ciliate protozoal numbers can vary from none in some unusual situations (SMITH & MCALLAN, 1974) to $>10^6$ depending on the composition of the diet and conditions within the rumen of the host animal (HUNGATE, 1966).

An *in vitro* system such as the one described here would be expected to maintain lower numbers of protozoa than would be found *in vivo* in the rumen because of a lowered feed input per unit volume of digesta and a relatively rapid turnover rate; generation time of protozoa can be as long as 3 days (CZERKAWSKI & BRECKENRIDGE, 1977).

In our experiments we followed HOOVER et al. (1976 a) in stirring intermittently. It has been suggested that continuous and vigorous mechanical agitation can adversely affect protozoal capacity for survical (NAKAMURA & KURIHARA, 1978; G. S. COLEMAN, personal communication). Certainly, protozoa survived well under the present conditions, and subsequently we have found that even with continuous stirring (100 rpm) numbers could be maintained in excess of 10^5/ml with other diets (R. J. MERRY & A. B. MCALLAN, unpublished observation). It seems likely that using a filtered outflow to retain feed particles leads to sequestration of protozoa in the vessel (ABE & KURIHARA, 1984). Recently these authors progressed further by adding an inert matrix to the culture vessel which encouraged sequestration and led to greater numbers and diversity of species, even under conditions of mechanical agitation and fairly low pH.

A distinct advantage of the system described is that solid feed is not restrained in a separate compartment within the vessel (WELLER & PILGRIM, 1974; CZERKAWSKI & BRECKENRIDGE, 1977), but enters continuously while digesta leaves, and does so in a manner which can be controlled to produce a variety of steady-state conditions. Our use of a relatively coarse filter mesh size compared with that used by earlier workers (e.g. STERN *et al.*, 1978) meant that filters did not have to be changed. Only small changes in effluent DM content were seen during the first few days and, after that, conditions remained remarkably constant. The main purpose of the filter is to control the passage of insoluble fibre from the vessel; and it is important that filtered effluent should contain little of this material. That this was achieved was indicated by the fact that little of the plant cell-wall sugars arabinose, xylose and cellulose-glucose were found in combined forms in filtered effluent. Starch-glucose was present in relatively greater amounts in filtered effluent but this must have been largely microbial in origin as the true digestibility of starch-glucose in the vessels was of the order of 98 % in these experiments.

The present results provided substantial confirmation of our preliminary finding that steady-state conditions can be achieved within 4–6 days in a system of the type described (MERRY et al., 1983). The plateau values for TVFA concentrations and pH in the vessels were within the accepted physiological range found in the rumens of cattle and sheep fed similar diets, and molar proportions of VFA's were also fairly typical for diets containing 50 % or more roughage (MURPHY et al., 1982). These findings were in contrast to those of some other authors who have observed concentrations of TVFA as high as 120–160 m mol/l (STERN, 1984; HANNAH et al., 1986). Such concentrations are not generally encountered *in vivo*, even 1–2 h post-feeding. Provision of a dialysis system (ABE & KUMENO, 1973) might permit a closer approach to *in vivo* turnover rates but would make the apparatus more complex. An alternative approach might be to control pH by addition of alkali (CRAWFORD et al., 1983), but would not prevent end-product accumulation.

Another objective of these experiments was to study the application of the nucleic acid-^{32}P incorporation method described by MERRY et al. (1982) to make estimates of microbial growth in the *in vitro* system. Values for daily flows of microbial nucleic acid-^{32}P reached equilibrium after 3–4 days infusion of $^{32}PO_4$ and, in agreement with measurements made for other indicators of microbial activity, were stable up to 19 days. Microbial N flows were estimated from effluent ^{32}P flows using values for the ratio nucleic acid $^{32}P/N$ in mixed bacteria harvested from the vessel contents. This value might be expected to be fairly constant where feeding is continuous, compared to twice a day feeding (SMITH & MCALLAN, 1974; CRAWFORD et al., 1980 b) where diurnal changes in the ratio RNA-N/total N were encountered. Although there were differences between experiments in absolute amounts of N and ^{32}P in bacterial cells the ratio remained fairly constant. There was also very little difference between nucleic acid-$^{32}P/N$ values in bacteria harvested from mixed effluent over a period of 24 h, and those harvested from vessel contents, suggesting that storage in ice for 24 h does not adversely affect bacterial cell composition. This finding will allow greater flexibility in future experiments. Observed values for TVFA and ammonia concentration, and protozoal numbers and pH are generally within the reported ranges of *in vivo* values taken from the literature. In addition the production of microbial N in relation to VFA production was compatible with reported *in vivo* values (SUTTON et al., 1970).

Summary

An *in vitro* continuous culture system to simulate processes in the rumen is described. This comprises a culture vessel (Fig. 2) fed continuously with pelleted solid feed (Fig. 1); artificial saliva also enters the vessel while effluent leaves it continuously in two streams, one is filtered and the other simply overflows (Fig. 1). In this way liquid and solid turnover times may be manipulated independently; in a trial experiment the former and latter were 6.3 % and 3.4 % per hour respectively.

In four replicated experiments a steady-state was achieved in 5–6 days with a feed of barley, tapioca, fishmeal, urea and straw and maintained for a further 7 to 14 days. During a steady-state period, rumen characteristics in terms of protozoal count, pH, redox potential, total volatile fatty acid concentration and ammonia concentration were stable and similar to those found in the rumens of animals given similar diets. Flows of microbial N compounds were assessed by infused $Na_2H^{32}PO_4$ with the artificial saliva and estimating the ^{32}P label incorporated in bacterial fractions.

The system demonstrably provided a satisfactory means for studying many aspects of rumen function.

Zusammenfassung

R. J. MERRY, R. H. SMITH und A. B. MCALLAN

Untersuchungen zur Pansenfunktion in einem kontinuierlichen *in-vitro*-Fermentationssystem

Es wird ein kontinuierliches *in-vitro*-Fermentationssystem zur Stimulierung von Pansenprozessen beschrieben. Dieses umfaßt ein Fermentationsgefäß (Abb. 2), das kontinuierlich mit pelletiertem festem Futter versorgt wird (Abb. 1). Ebenfalls wird dem Gefäß künstlicher Speichel zugeführt, während der Abfluß es in 2 Strömen verläßt, der eine ist gefiltert und der andere fließt einfach über (Abb. 1). Auf diese Weise können die Turnover-Zeiteinheiten der flüssigen und festen Phase unabhängig voneinander manipuliert werden; in einem Versuch betrugen sie 6,3 % für die erstere bzw. 3,4 % pro h für letztere Fraktion. In 4 Wiederholungsexperimenten wurde für eine Futtermischung aus Gerste, Tapioka, Fischmehl, Harnstoff und Stroh in 5–6 Tagen ein Gleichgewichtszustand erreicht, das weitere 7–14 Tage aufrecht erhalten werden konnte. Während einer Gleichgewichtsperiode waren die Pansen-Charakteristika in der Protozoenanzahl, im pH-Wert, im Redoxpotential, in der Konzentration an flüchtigen Fettsäuren und Ammoniak stabil und ähnlich den Verhältnissen im Pansen, wenn die Tiere analoge Diäten erhielten. Der Fluß von mikrobiellen N-Verbindungen wurde mittels infundiertem $NaH_2{}^{32}PO_4$ über den künstlichen Speichel und der Bestimmung der ^{32}P-Inkorporation in bakterielle Fraktionen gemessen.

Das System ist nachweislich so ausgerüstet, daß es befriedigende Werte zum Studium vieler Aspekte der Pansenfunktion liefert.

Резюме

Р. И. Мерри, Р. Х. Смис и А. Б. МэкЭллен

Исследование по работе рубца в постоянной системе ферментации *in vitro*

Описывается постоянная система ферментации *in vitro* для моделирования рубцовых процессов. Она состоит из ферментационного прибора (см. рис. 2), в который постоянно введётся гранулированный твёрдый корм (см. рис. 1). Кроме того введётся в прибор искусственная слюна, а выделение из прибора происходит двумя путями, один поток фильтруется и другой только так перетечёт (см. рис. 1). Таким образом можно манипулировать переходные времени (*Turnover*) жидкой и твёрдой фаз независимо друг от друга; в одном опыте они были 6,3 %/h для жидкой фазы и 3,4 %/час для твёрдой фракции. С помощью 4 повторных экспериментов с применением кормовой смеси из ячменя, тапиоки, рыбной муки, мочевины и соломы получено через 5–6 дней состояние равновесия, которое содержалось ещё 7–14 дней. Во время периода равновесия параметры рубца как число простейших, pH, окислительно-восстановительный потенциал, концентрация летучих жирных кислот и аммиака являлись стабильными и похожими состояния в рубце, если животные получили аналогичные диеты. Течение микробных азотистых соединений определилось с помощью инфундированного $NaH_2{}^{32}PO_4$ в искусственной слюне и с помощью включения ^{32}P в бактериальные фракции. Доказывали, что система даёт удовлетворяемые результаты для учёбы многоразных аспектов работы рубца.

References

[1] ABE, M. and F. KUMENO: J. Anim. Sci. **36**, 941 (1973)
[2] ABE, M. and Y. KURIHARA: J. Appl. Bact. **56**, 201 (1984)
[3] AGRICULTURAL RESEARCH COUNCIL: The Nutrient Requirements of Farm Livestock. Commonwealth Agricultural Bureaux, Slough (1980)

[4] CRAWFORD, R. J., W. H. HOOVER and P. H. KNOWLTON: J. Anim. Sci. **51**, 975 (1980 a)
[5] CRAWFORD, R. J., W. H. HOOVER and L. L. JUNKINS: J. Anim. Sci. **51**, 986 (1980 b)
[6] CRAWFORD, R. J., B. J. SHRIVER, G. A. VARGA and W. H. HOOVER: J. Dairy Sci. **66**, 1881 (1983)
[7] CZERKAWSKI, J. W.: Laboratory Practice, **25**, 17 (1976)
[8) CZERKAWSKI, J. W.: In 'An Introduction to Rumen Studies', 236 p. Oxford: Pergamon press (1986)
[9] CZERKAWSKI, J. W. and G. BRECKENRIDGE: Brit. J. Nutrit. **38**, 371 (1977)
[10] DAVEY, L. A., G. C. CHEESEMAN and C. A. E. BRIGGS: J. Agric. Sci., Camb. **55**, 155 (1966)
[11] EWART, J. M.: Proc. Nutrit. Soc. **33**, 125 (1974)
[12] HANNAH, S. M., STERN, M. D. and F. R. EHLE: Anim. Feed Sci. Technol. **16**, 51 (1986)
[13] HOBSON, P. N.: J. Gen. Microbiol. **38**, 161 (1965)
[14] HOOVER, W. H., B. A. CROOKER and C. J. SNIFFEN: J. Anim. Sci. **43**, 528 (1976 a)
[15] HOOVER, W. H., R. H. KNOWLTON, M. D. STERN and C. J. SNIFFEN: J. Anim. Sci. **43**, 535 (1976 b)
[16] HUNGATE, R. E.: The Rumen and its Microbes, New York, Academic Press (1966)
[17] M. A. F. F. Energy Allowances and Feeding Systems for Ruminants, Technical Bulletin 33, London. HMSO (1975)
[18] McDOUGALL, E. I. Biochem. J. **43**, 99 (1948)
[19] MERRY, R. J.: The use of dietary non-protein nitrogen compounds by the ruminant with particular emphasis on the glycosyl ureides. Ph. D. Thesis, University of Reading (1980)
[20] MERRY, R. J., A. B. McALLAN and R. H. SMITH: Brit. J. Nutrit. **48**, 287 (1982)
[21] MERRY, R. J., R. H. SMITH and A. B. McALLAN: In: Protein Metabolism and Nutrition, pp. 227–230 (R. PION, M. ARNAL and D. BONIN, editors), Paris: INRA (1983)
[22] MERRY, R. J., R. H. SMITH and A. B. McALLAN: Proc. Nutrit. Soc. 43, 34 A (1984 a)
[23] MERRY, R. J., R. H. SMITH and A. B. McALLAN: Can. J. Anim. Sci. 64, (Supplement), 56 (1984 b)
[24] McALLAN, A. B. and R. H. SMITH: Brit. J. Nutrit. 23, 671 (1969)
[25] McALLAN, A. B. and R. H. SMITH: Brit. J. Nutrit. **31**, 77 (1974)
[26] MURPHY, M. R., R. L. BALDWIN and M. J. KOONG: J. Anim. Sci. 55, 411 (1982)
[27] NAKAMURA, F. and Y. KURIHARA: Appl. Environ. Microbiol. **35**, 500 (1978)
[28] RUFENER, W. H., W. O. NELSON and M. J. WOLIN: Appl. Microbiol. **11**, 196 (1963)
[29] SLYTER, L. L., W. O. NELSON and M. J. WOLIN: Appl. Microbiol. **12**, 374 (1964)
[30] SMITH, R. H. and A. B. McALLAN: Brit. J. Nutrit. **24**, 545 (1970)
[31] SMITH, R. H. and A. B. McALLAN: Brit. J. Nutrit. **31**, 27 (1974)
[32] SMITH, R. H., A. B. McALLAN, D. HEWITT and P. E. LEWIS: J. Agric. Sci. Camb. **90**, 557 (1978)
[33] STERN, M. D.: Can. J. Anim. Sci. **64** (Supplement), 27 (1984)
[34] STERN, M. D., W. H. HOOVER, C. J. SNIFFEN, B. A. CROOKER and P. H. KNOWLTON: J. Anim. Sci. **47**, 944 (1978)
[35] SUTTON, J. D., T. SMITH and D. A. CORSE.: In: Energy Metabolism of Farm Animals. EAAP Publication No. 13, Zürich (in Druck)
[36] WELLER, R. A. and A. F. PILGRIM: Brit. J. Nutrit. **32**, 341 (1974)

Acknowledgements

The authors would like to thank Dr J. W. SISSONS, Mr. A. R. JONES and Mrs C. JONES and staff for care of the animals and Dr D. Hewitt for advice on statistical treatment. They are also grateful to Mr E. S. GRIFFITH, Mr A. WOODHOUSE and Miss C. RUMNEY for skilled technical assistance. The National Institute for Research in Dairying now forms constituent parts of the Animal and Grassland Research Institute and the Food Research Institute, Reading Laboratory and was financed through the Agricultural and Food Research Council; the work in part commissioned by the Ministry of Agriculture, Fisheries and Food.

Received 6 January 1987

Addresses of authors:

Dr. R. J. MERRY and Dr. A. B. MCALLAN
Present addresses:
Animal and Grassland Research Institute, Hurley, Maidenhead,
Berks, SL6 5LR
UK

Dr. R. H. SMITH
c/o Animal and Grassland Research Institute, Shinfield, Reading, RG2 9AQ
UK

Arch. Anim. Nutr., Berlin 37 (1987) 6, 489–503

Institut für Ernährungsphysiologie der Technischen Universität München

M. Kreuzer und M. Kirchgessner

Untersuchungen zur nutritiven Defaunierung des Pansens beim Wiederkäuer

1. Einleitung

Defaunierung, die selektive Abtötung der tierischen Mikroben bei Erhaltung der bakteriellen Aktivität im Pansen, scheint unter bestimmten Bedingungen vorteilhaft für Wachstum und Futterverwertung beim Wiederkäuer zu sein (vgl. Literaturzusammenstellungen bei Kreuzer, 1986, Leinmüller und Menke, 1986 sowie Veira, 1986). Dabei kann sowohl der Ansatz an Protein (Klopfenstein u. a. 1966; Males und Purser, 1970; Takahashi und Kametaka, 1976; Kreuzer und Kirchgessner, 1986) als auch an Energie (Whitelaw u. a., 1984; Kreuzer u. a., 1986) erhöht sein. Methoden, bei denen die Fauna mit oberflächenaktiven Substanzen (Terics, Manoxol, Alkanat) abgetötet wird, sind umstritten und schwierig durchzuführen (Eadie und Shand, 1981; Lovelock u. a., 1982), so daß sie allenfalls für experimentelle Zwecke geeignet sind. Dies gilt auch für eine Methode, bei der der Panseninhalt entleert und anschließend der Pansen desinfiziert wird (Jouany und Senaud, 1979). Soll die positive Wirkung der Defaunierung auf die Fütterungspraxis übertragen werden, so sind physiologische Methoden nötig, die zudem keine größeren Leistungseinbrüche durch die Prozedur der Defaunierung per se zur Folge haben. Dies könnte durch die sogenannte nutritive Defaunierung erfolgen, also eine Defaunierung mit Ernährungsmaßnahmen. In der Literatur wurde bereits vor längerer Zeit beschrieben, wie der Wiederkäuer seine Protozoen als Folge der angewandten Fütterungsweise verlieren kann, nämlich durch ad lib. vorgelegtes, pelletiertes, konzentriertes Futter (Christiansen u. a., 1964; Eadie u. a., 1967) oder durch Milch (Eberlein, 1895). In der vorliegenden Untersuchung sollte geprüft werden, inwieweit diese Ansätze zu praktisch anwendbaren Defaunierungsmethoden weiterentwickelt werden können. Zudem sollten Anhaltspunkte für die jeweils zugrundeliegenden Wirkungsmechanismen gewonnen werden.

2. Material und Methodik

Die Defaunierung mit Kraftfutter und Milch wurde *in vitro* und *in vivo* (an Lämmern und Färsen) erprobt. Dabei wurden jeweils in empirisch festgelegten Zeitabständen Pansensaftproben gezogen. Im geseihten Pansensaft wurde sodann der pH-Wert gemessen und die Einflüsse auf die Protozoenpopulation mit folgenden Abstufungen bewertet: unverändert (=), erhöht (>), erniedrigt (<) und defauniert (0). Die Zu-

Tabelle 1 (Table 1)
Zusammensetzung der zur nutritiven Defaunierung eingesetzten Kraftfuttermischungen (Composition of the concentrates used for nutritive defaunation)

	Kraftfutter I (Concentrate I)	Kraftfutter II[1] (Concentrate II)
Komponenten (*Components*)		
	85 % Gerste[2] (Barley)	37,5 % Ackerbohnen (Horse beans)
	15 % Sojaextraktionsschrot (Soya bean meal)	22,5 % Maniok (Cassava)
		22,5 % Haferschälkleie (Oat huller feed)
		15,0 % Melasse (Molasses)
		2,3 % Mineralstoffmischung (Mineral mix)
		0,2 % $NaHCO_3$
Inhaltsstoffe (*Nutrient contents*)		
	90,6 % Trockensubstanz (DM)	88,7 % Trockensubstanz (DM)
	18,2 % Rohprotein (CP)	15,6 % Rohprotein (CP)
	4,8 % Rohfaser (CF)	9,6 % Rohfaser (CF)

[1] aus einem vorangegangenen Lämmerversuch übernommen (KREUZER und KIRCHGESSNER, 1987) (Taken from a preliminary lamb trial (KREUZER and KIRCHGESSNER, 1987))
[2] *in vitro* alternativ zu Gerste auch Mais, Weizen und Hafer (*In vitro* also corn, wheat and oats instead of barley used)

sammensetzung der verwendeten pelletierten Kraftfuttermischungen ist in Tab. 1 angegeben.

In den *in-vivo*-Experimenten wurden insgesamt 5 Färsen (260–400 kg Lebendmasse) und 14 Mastlämmer beiderlei Geschlechts (32–37 kg) eingesetzt. Das Kraftfutter wurde jeweils auf den blanken Trog verabreicht und es wurde verhindert, daß die Tiere Einstreu aufnahmen. Die Milch (Vollmilch mit etwa 4 % Fett) bzw. frische Sahne (30 % Fett) wurde hingegen über Flaschen eingeflößt und die Tiere erhielten keinerlei anderes Futter. Vor Verabreichung des jeweiligen Defaunierungsfutters wurden die Tiere eine Mahlzeit lang genüchtert. Sofort nach erfolgreicher Defaunierung bzw. nach Abbruch der Behandlung wurde wieder mit der Fütterung begonnen. Nach der Verabreichung großer Mengen Kraftfutter wurde zunächst nur Heu vorgelegt, bis die Tiere wieder eine normale Futteraufnahme zeigten. In allen *in-vivo*-Experimenten wurde der Pansensaft zur Analyse mit Hilfe von Schlundsonden gewonnen.

Die *in-vitro*-Experimente wurden mit Pansensaft und Puffermedium (1 : 2) nach der Methode von MENKE u. a. (1979) ausgeführt. Dabei wurden die zu untersuchenden Substanzen jeweils zu Beginn des Experiments auf einmal zugesetzt. Die Menge an Zusatz wurde dabei immer in % Anteilen am eingesetzten Pansensaft (ohne Puffermedium) bemessen. Kraftfutter bzw. Kraftfutterbestandteile wurden vorher grob gemahlen. Milchbestandteile, die nur in Pulverform vorrätig waren (Magermilch, teilentzuckerte Molke, Kasein, Laktose), wurden vor der Zugabe zum Pansensaft mit Wasser in Konzentrationen angerührt, die in etwa ihrem Gehalt in durchschnittlicher Vollmilch entsprachen. In den Versuchen mit Säurezusatz wurde ein Medium verwendet, das kein Natriumbikarbonat enthielt, ansonsten aber der Zusammensetzung des Puffermediums entsprach. Mit Ausnahme der Vollmilch, die bereits durch jeweils zwei ähnliche Proben vertreten war, wurden bei jedem Zusatz Doppelbestimmungen durchgeführt. Die in den Versuchen verwendeten Kolbenpipetten ermöglichten eine mehrmalige Probennahme ohne Störung des Gärverlaufs. Der Pansensaft für die *in-vitro*-Versuche wurde von fistulierten Hammeln gewonnen, die eine konventionelle Heu-Kraftfutterration erhielten.

3. Ergebnisse

Tabelle 2 gibt die *in-vivo*-Ergebnisse zur Defaunierung mit Kraftfutter an. Kraftfutter I war bei Lämmern deutlich wirksamer als Kraftfutter II. Bei der ad-lib.-Verfütterung der Gerste-Soja-Pellets waren nach 6 Stunden bereits zwei der drei Tiere protozoenfrei, während sich die Fauna beim rohfaserreicheren Kraftfutter II nach eintägiger ad-lib.-Fütterung nahezu unverändert zeigte.

Die unbegrenzte Vorlage von Kraftfutter I führte auch bei Färsen sicher zur Defaunierung. Im Gegensatz zu den Versuchen an Lämmern traten bei den Färsen jedoch

Tabelle 2 (Table 2)
Nutritive Defaunierung mit Kraftfutter *in vivo* (Nutritive defaunation with concentrate *in vivo*)

Tierart (Lambs or heifers)	Kraftfutter (Concentrate)	Konsistenz (Pellets or meal)	Menge[1], kg (Amount, kg)	Vorlagefrequenz (Feeding frequency)	1. Messung (1. measurement)			2. Messung (2. measurement)			3. Messung (3. measurement)		
					h[2]	P.[3]	pH	h	P.	pH	h	P.	pH
Lämmer (Lambs)	I	Pellets	a. l.	1 x	6	0	5,7						
	I	Pellets	a. l.	1 x	6	0	5,4						
	I	Pellets	a. l.	1 x	6	>	5,4	24	>	6,7			
	II	Pellets	a. l.	1 x	24	<	5,7						
	II	Pellets	a. l.	1 x	24	=	5,7						
	II	Pellets	a. l.	1 x	24	=	6,0						
	II	Pellets	a. l.	1 x	24	=	6,7						
Färsen (Heifers)	I	Pellets	8,5 a. l.	1 x	24	0	4,5	48	0	4,8	144	0	6,5
	I	Pellets	8,1 a. l.	1 x	17	0	4,3	22	0	4,5	168	0	7,4
	I	Pellets	3,6 res.	4 x	4	=	7,0	8	<	7,0	168	=	7,0
	I	Pellets	4,0 res.	1 x	1	=	7,0	5	=	7,0	168	=	7,0
	I	Pellets	5,8 res.	1 x	5	=	6,7	8	<	5,7	24	0	4,1
	I	Mehl	a. l.	1 x	24	>	6,2	48	=	7,5			

[1]a. l. = ad-libitum-Vorlage; res. = restriktive Vorlage (a. l. = ad libitum feeding; res. = restrictive feeding)
[2]h = Stunden nach Beginn der Kraftfuttervorlage (h = hours after feeding concentrate)
[3]p. = Protozoenzahl; = : unverändert; > : erhöht; < : erniedrigt; 0: defauniert
(P. = Protozoal counts; = : not varied; > : higher; < : lower, 0: defaunated)

ernsthafte gesundheitliche Probleme auf. Die sehr tiefen pH-Werte von 4,3–4,5 im Vergleich zu 5,4–5,7 bei den Lämmern deuten auf eine schwere Pansenazidose hin. Tatsächlich wiesen die Tiere über kurze Zeit einige Symptome dafür auf, nämlich Inappetenz, Durchfall, Muskelzittern und leichtes Festliegen. Die Therapie mit größeren Mengen temperierter Pufferlösung, die eingeflößt wurde, und mit der Vorlage von gutem Heu erbrachte jedoch schnell eine Besserung des Zustandes. Um das Azidoserisiko zu mindern, wurde versucht, die Kraftfuttergaben aufzuteilen (stündlich je 1 kg) bzw. das Kraftfutter restriktiv vorzulegen (Tab. 2). Die Aufteilung der Kraftfuttergabe führte nicht zum Erfolg, ebensowenig wie die Vorlage von 4 kg Kraftfutter auf einmal. Wurden jedoch 6 kg Kraftfutter auf einmal vorgelegt, so trat mit einer Verzögerung von über 8 Stunden eine drastische Wirkung auf (Tab. 2). Der pH-Wert erreichte dabei eher ein noch tieferes Niveau als bei ad-lib.-Fütterung, obwohl das hier eingesetzte Tier im Gegensatz zu den anderen 14 Tage lang genau an dieses Kraftfutter mit 1 kg/d adaptiert worden war. Ein Versuch, die Defaunierung mit unpelletiertem, mehlförmigem Kraftfutter zu erreichen, führte nicht zum Erfolg.

Die Ergebnisse aus den *in-vitro*-Versuchen mit Kraftfutter sind in Tab. 3 wiedergegeben. In den Kontrollansätzen war die Protozoenpopulation nach 48 Stunden etwas reduziert, aber noch eindeutig vital. Bei der Zulage von Kraftfutter war der Pansensaft dagegen spätestens nach einem Tag protozoenfrei und der pH-Wert lag um etwa 2 Einheiten unter den Kontrollwerten. Wurde die Gerste in Kraftfutter I durch andere Getreidearten ersetzt, so zeigte sich bei Weizen eine etwas schnellere Wirkung gegen

Tabelle 3 (Table 3)

Nutritive Defaunierung mit Kraftfutter (KF) *in vitro* in Abhängigkeit von Menge und Art an Zusatz (Nutritive defaunation with concentrate *in vitro* in relation to kind and amout of supplementation)

Zusatz (Supplement)	Anteil, % (Portion, %)	maximale Zeit bis zur Defaunierung, h (Maximum time till defaunation, h)	End-pH (Final pH)
kein Zusatz (No supplement)	0	>48	7,0
KF I/Gerste (Conc. I/barley)	10	21	5,4
	20	8	4,9
	30	6	5,1
	40[1]	8	4,9
KF I/Weizen (Wheat)	10	19	5,4
KF I/Mais (Corn)	10	23	5,4
KF I/Hafer (Oats)	10	24	5,4
Weizenstärke (Wheat starch)	10	21	5,4
Maisstärke (Corn starch)	10	23	5,4
KF II (Concentrate II)	20	24	5,0
	40	8	4,3

[1] Benetzung mit Pansensaft nicht vollständig möglich (Complete moistening with rumen fluid not possible)

Protozoen, bei Mais und Hafer dauerte es dagegen etwas länger bis zur Defaunierung. Bei Einsatz von Mais war zudem zu beobachten, daß der pH-Wert länger hoch blieb als bei den übrigen Getreidearten, dann aber sehr schnell abfiel. Wurde reine Stärke (Weizen, Mais) ohne Proteinsupplement zugelegt, so ergaben sich vergleichbare Wirkungen. Aus Tabelle 3 wird außerdem deutlich, daß das Gerste-Soja-Kraftfutter (I) schneller und stärker wirkte als das rohfaserreichere Kraftfutter (II), wie schon *in vivo* zu beobachten war.

In weiteren *in-vitro*-Versuchen wurde der Bedeutung der Rohfaser bzw. einzelner Faserbestandteile bei der nutritiven Defaunierung nachgegangen (Tab. 4). Heu verzögerte die Wirkung gegen Protozoen deutlich. Dieser Effekt scheint vor allem auf die

Tabelle 4 (Table 4)

Verzögerung der nutritiven Defaunierung mit Kraftfutter durch Rauhfutter bzw. verschiedene Faserbestandteile *in vitro* (Delay of nutritive defaunation with concentrate by additional roughage or different kinds of fibre *in vitro*)

Zusatz an Kraftfutter (Addition of concentrate)	Zusatz an Rohfaser (Addition of crude fibre)	maximale Zeit bis zur Defaunierung, h (Maximum time till defaunation, h)	End-pH (Final pH)
–	–	>48	7,0
30 % KF I (Conc. I)	–	6	5,1
25 % KF I (Conc. I)	5 % Heu (Hay)	24	5,2
10 % Weizenstärke (Wheat starch)	–	21	5,4
7,5 % "	2,5 % Zellulose (Cellulose)	31	5,2
5,0 % "	5,0 % Zellulose (Cellulose)	>48	5,4
–	10 % Zellulose (Cellulose)	>48	5,6
7,5 % "	2,5 % Lignin (Lignin)	28	5,2
5,0 % "	5,0 % Lignin (Lignin)	>48	5,3
–	10 % Lignin (Lignin)	>48	6,9
7,5 % "	2,5 % Pektin (Pectin)	24	5,0
5,0 % "	5,0 % Pektin (Pectin)	25	5,0
–	10 % Pektin (Pectin)	(25)[1]	4,9
7,5 % "	2,5 % Xylose (Xylose)	24	4,7
5,0 % "	5,0 % Xylose (Xylose)	24	5,1
–	10 % Xylose (Xylose)	24	5,1

[1] Probe geliert (Sample gelatinized)

darin enthaltene Zellulose und auch auf das Lignin zurückzuführen zu sein, wohingegen Pektin und Xylose (stellvertretend für Hemizellulosen) keine Verzögerung bewirkten. Bei Zusatz von 0,2 bis 10 % Natriumbikarbonat oder von 3 % Mineralfutter zu Kraftfutter I ergaben sich keine Unterschiede in der Zeitspanne bis zur Defaunierung.

Da der pH-Wert in allen Versuchen mit Zulagen von Kraftfutter deutlich absank, bevor die Defaunierung eintrat, wurde der Effekt von Säuren gegen Protozoen untersucht (Tab. 5). Dazu wurde neben Schwefelsäure auch Milchsäure verwendet, die bei hoher Kraftfutteraufnahme im Pansen auftritt. Bei Zusatz von Milchsäure starben die Protozoen bereits bei pH-Werten von 4,7–4,8 augenblicklich ab, während dies mit

Tabelle 5 (Table 5)
Wirkung einer Absenkung des pH-Wertes mit Schwefelsäure und Milchsäure *in vitro* auf die Pansenfauna (Effects of lowering pH by sulfuric and lactic acid *in vitro* on rumen protozoa)

Anfangs-pH[1] (Initial pH)	Schwefelsäure End-pH (Sulfuric acid) (Final pH)	max. Zeit bis zur Defaunierung (Maximum time till defaunation)	Milchsäure End-pH (Lactic acid) (Final pH)	max. Zeit bis zur Defaunierung (Maximum time till defaunation)
4,3	4,3	0	4,3	0
4,4	4,4	0–1	4,4	0
4,5	4,6	1–2	4,5	0
4,6	4,6	1	4,6	0
4,7	4,7	1	4,7	0
4,8	4,8	1–2	4,8	0–0,5
4,9	5,0	1–2	5,0	1–2
5,0	5,0	5–6	5,0	4–5
5,1	5,2	9	5,2	8
5,2	5,4	<24[2]	5,2	8
5,3	5,4	<24	5,8	<24[2]
5,4	5,5	<24	5,8	<24
5,5	5,6	<24	5,7	<24
6,0	6,0	>24	5,8	>24

[1] mit der jeweiligen Säure eingestellt; Medium ohne Pufferzusatz (Adapted with the respective acid; medium without buffer)
[2] keine Messung zwischen 9 und 24 h (No measurement between 9 and 24 h)

Schwefelsäure erst bei pH 4,3–4,4 der Fall war. Bei pH-Werten um 5,0 lag noch eine intensive Wirkung gegen Protozoen vor, bei höheren pH-Werten dauerte es deutlich länger, bis die Protozoen *in vitro* abstarben. Die Unterschiede in der Wirkung von Schwefelsäure und Milchsäure wurden mit steigenden pH-Werten geringer.

Die Ergebnisse zum *in-vivo*-Effekt von Milch auf die Pansenfauna sind in Tabelle 6 zusammengestellt. Bei Lämmern konnten 3 von 7 Tieren bereits durch eine einmalige Gabe von 300 ml Vollmilch defauniert werden, weitere zwei Lämmer waren nach einer zweiten, um 24 Stunden vesetzten Gabe von 300 ml protozoenfrei, obwohl etwa eine Stunde nach der zweiten Gabe wieder mit der normalen Fütterung begonnen worden war. Der pH-Wert im Pansensaft lag bei Lämmern und Färsen kurz nach der Milchfütterung relativ hoch. Der im Anschluß aufgetretene pH-Abfall im Pansensaft der Lämmer in den Tagen nach der Milchzufuhr ist auf die wieder verabreichte kraftfutterreiche Mastration zurückzuführen. Im Gegensatz zu den Lämmern konnte bei Färsen keine Defaunierung durch Vollmilch erzielt werden, wenn auch die Protozoenzahl jeweils nach 24 Stunden verringert war (Tab. 6). Eine Defaunierung wurde auch nicht erreicht, wenn die Milchmenge von 2 auf 4 Liter erhöht wurde oder wenn insgesamt 6 Liter in Literportionen auf zwei Tage verteilt eingegeben wurden. Höhere Mengen wurden wegen der steigenden Gefahr von Pansenfäule aufgrund hoher Mengen an Milcheiweiß nicht verabreicht. Hingegen wurde die Fauna durch das Einflößen von einem Liter frischer Sahne (äquivalent zu 7,5 Litern Vollmilch) schnell und problemlos abgetötet.

Tabelle 6 (Table 6)

Nutritive Defaunierung mit Milch *in vivo* (Nutritive defaunation with milk *in vivo*)

Tierart (Lambs or heifers)	Milchmenge ml 1. Anwend. (Milk 1. application) (ml)	Milchmenge wiederh. Anw. nach h (Milk, repeated application) (after h)	ml (ml)	1. Messung (1. measurement) h[1]	P.[2]	pH	2. Messung (2. measurement) h	P.	pH	3. Messung (3. measurement) h	P.	pH
Lämmer (Lambs)	300			24	0	7,0	168	0	5,7			
	300			24	0	7,0	168	0	5,7			
	300			24	0	7,0	48	0	6,4			
	300	24	300	24	<	7,0	48	0	6,2			
	300	24	300	24	=	7,0	48	0	6,4	168	<	5,7
	300	24	300	24	<	7,0	48	<	6,7			
	300	24	300	24	<	7,0	48	<	6,4			
Färsen (Heifers)	2000			8	=	7,0	24	<	7,0	48	=	7,0
	4000			24	<	7,0	48	=	7,0			
	1000	4	1000									
		9	1000									
		24	1000									
		28	1000									
		33	1000	48	=	7,0						
	1000[3]			8	0	7,0	30	0	7,0			

[1] h = Stunden nach Beginn der Milcheingabe (h = hours after milk application)

[2] P. = Protozoenzahl; = : unverändert; > : erhöht; < : erniedrigt; 0 = defauniert (P. = Protozoal counts; = : not varied; > : higher; < : lower; 0 = defaunated)

[3] frische Sahne mit 30 % Fett, fettäquivalent zu 7,5 l Vollmilch mit 4 % Fett (Fresh cream containing 30 % fat; equivalent in fat to 7,5 l whole milk with 4 % fat)

Tab. 7 zeigt die Ergebnisse der *in-vitro*-Defaunierung mit Milch verschiedenen Fettgehalts. Die Ergebnisse legen den Schluß nahe, daß der Milchbestandteil Fett für die defaunierende Wirkung der Milch verantwortlich sein könnte, da mit steigendem Fettgehalt des Zusatzes schneller ein Effekt gegen Protozoen auftrat bzw. schon eine geringere Menge zum gewünschten Ergebnis führte.

Um diese Vermutung zu überprüfen, wurde die Wirkung der anderen quantitativen Milchbestandteile auf die Protozoen in möglichst isolierter Form untersucht. Dazu wurden ebenfalls steigende Mengen verwendet (2, 5, 10 und 50 % Anteil am eingesetzten Pansensaft). Laktose, Kasein und teilentzuckerte Molke zeigten auch bei der höchsten Zulagestufe noch nach 48 Stunden keine meßbare Wirkung auf die Protozoen. Auch der pH-Wert (6,4–7,0) veränderte sich im Vergleich zum Kontrollansatz nur wenig. Außerdem wurde die Wirkung von Fett anderer Herkunft auf die Protozoen überprüft, und zwar so, daß die gleiche Menge Fett wie im Falle der Sahne (Tab. 7) zugesetzt wurde. Eine Suspension von Sojaöl in Wasser hatte keine Wirkung, wohl da eine schnelle Entmischung stattfand und so die Kontaminationsmöglichkeit mit den Mikroben gering war. Dagegen ergaben sich durch ein emulgiertes Fett („Micafett 60"; 36 % Tierfett, 18 % gehärtetes Seetieröl, 6 % Pflanzenfett, 35 % Laktose, 5 % Kasein) Effekte gegen Protozoen. Die Fauna wurde jedoch erst nach 48 Stunden abge-

Tabelle 7 (Table 7)

Nutritive Defaunierung mit Milch *in vitro* (Nutritive defaunation with milk *in vitro*)

Milchtyp (Kind of milk)	Fettgehalt, % (Fat content, %)	Anteil der Milch, % (Portion of milk, %)	maximale Zeit bis zur Defaunierung, h (Maximum time till defaunation, h)	End-pH (Final pH)
kein Zusatz (No supplement)	–	0	>48	7,0
Magermilch (Skim milk)	<0,5	2	>48	6,7
	<0,5	5	>48	6,7
	<0,5	10	>48	6,7
	<0,5	50	>48	6,7
Vollmilch (Whole milk)	3,5	5	>48	6,7
	3,5	10	48	7,3
	3,5	15	48	6,7
Vollmilch (Whole milk)	3,9	8	48	6,7
	3,9	10	>48	6,7
	3,9	12	48	6,7
	3,9	20	31	6,7
Vollmilch (Whole milk)	5,9	1	>27	7,2
	5,9	5	>27	7,2
	5,9	20	26	7,0
	5,9	50	24	5,5
Vollmilch (Whole milk)	6,2	5	48	7,5
	6,2	10	48	6,8
	6,2	15	28	7,1
Kondensmilch (Evaporated milk)	12	5	>48	7,1
	12	10	24	6,7
	12	15	24	6.6
Sahne (Cream)	30	5	24	6,7
	30	10	24	6,7
	30	15	24	6,6

tötet und dies auch nur bei einem Zusatz von mindestens 10 %. Die Wirkung fiel also deutlich schwächer aus als bei frischer Sahne. Zudem ging der pH-Wert umso stärker zurück, je höher die Dosierung war (5 %: 6,2; 10 %: 6,0; 15 %: 5,6). Tabelle 7 verdeutlicht, daß die Defaunierung mit Milch dagegen weitgehend ohne Einfluß auf den pH-Wert blieb, wie es auch *in vivo* der Fall war. Im Vergleich zu den *in-vitro*-Versuchen mit Kraftfutter wird aber offenbar, daß Milch doch deutlich schwächer bzw. langsamer gegen Protozoen wirkt.

4. Diskussion

Nutritive Methoden zur Defaunierung wurden bisher kaum beachtet, möglicherweise da chemische Methoden für experimentelle Zwecke einfach und zuverlässig genug erschienen. Für die praktische Anwendung sind diese im Gegensatz zu den nutritiven Methoden jedoch kaum brauchbar, da die Applikation über Schlundsonden schwierig ist und Risiken bezüglich der Tiergesundheit vorliegen. Chemikalienrückstände in den

Verkaufsprodukten sind zwar nicht sehr wahrscheinlich, können aber nicht ausgeschlossen werden. Werden jedoch nutritive Methoden angewandt, so entfällt einmal das Rückstandsproblem und andererseits kann möglicherweise der Wachstumsknick als Folge der Defaunierungsprozedur vermindert oder gar vermieden werden. Bei den chemischen Methoden ergibt sich dieser Wachstumsknick durch die notwendige Nüchterung vor und nach der Applikation des Mittels (ORPIN, 1977) sowie durch einen Rückgang des Appetits aufgrund der Detergentien selbst, so daß der erwartete Wachstumsvorteil der defaunierten Tiere möglicherweise nur ausreicht, diesen Einbruch auszugleichen (BURGGRAAF, 1980). In der vorliegenden Arbeit wurden zwei erfolgversprechende nutritive Methoden getestet.

4.1. Defaunierung durch Kraftfutter

Nach JOHNSON (1976) ist es in der Praxis, besonders bei intensiver Kraftfuttermast, gar nicht so ungewöhnlich, protozoenfreie Wiederkäuer aufzufinden. Dies bestätigte sich in einem vor kurzem abgeschlossenen Versuch an Lämmern (KREUZER und KIRCHGESSNER, 1987), in dem alle Tiere der Gruppe mit der höchsten Energieaufnahme zu Mastende protozoenfrei waren, obwohl auch 150 g/d Heu zugefüttert wurde. Bei Verfütterung eines anderen Kraftfutters (identisch mit Kraftfutter II, Tab. 1) mit niedrigerer Energieaufnahme waren dagegen durchwegs Protozoen im Pansen der Tiere vorhanden. Mit steigendem Kraftfutteranteil in der Ration erhöht sich zunächst die Zahl der Protozoen, geht aber dann bei sehr hohen Anteilen drastisch zurück (MACKIE u. a., 1978). Werden alle Rationskomponenten (Grund- und Kraftfutter) ad lib. und pelletiert vorgelegt, so ist zu erwarten, daß die Protozoenzahl nach spätestens 2–3 Wochen auf Null zurückgeht (CHRISTIANSEN u. a., 1964). EADIE u. a. (1967) entwickelten aus Beobachtungen bei der Verfütterung eines pelletierten Kraftfutters mit 85 % Gerste und 15 % Proteinkonzentrat an Bullen eine Defaunierungsmethode, die später routinemäßig in Experimenten der gleichen Arbeitsgruppe zur Anwendung kam (WHITELAW u. a., 1972 und 1984). Wurde dieses Kraftfutter ad lib. vorgelegt, so waren die Tiere (hier Bullen und Färsen) nach 1–2 Tagen protozoenfrei, wurde die Aufnahme aber auf unter 75 % der freiwilligen Aufnahme restriktiert, so ergab sich kein Effekt (EADIE u. a., 1970).

Im vorliegenden Experiment wurde mit dem Kraftfutter I eine Mischung eingesetzt, die dem Kraftfutter von EADIE u. a. (1967) weitgehend entsprach. Es bestätigte sich, daß relativ hohe Mengen Kraftfutter nötig sind, um die Protozoen abzutöten. Bei Färsen scheint jedoch nicht unbedingt eine ad-lib.-Zufuhr nötig zu sein. So reichten bereits 78 g Kraftfutter je kg $LM^{0,75}$, also etwa 85 % der freiwilligen Aufnahme (90 bis 95 $g/kg^{0,75}$), zur Defaunierung aus, nicht jedoch 54 g (Tab. 2 : 4,0 kg Kraftfutter I). Die ad-lib.-Aufnahme des Gerste-Proteinsupplements lag in den Versuchen von EADIE u. a. (1970) und WHITELAW u. a. (1972 und 1984) mit 87–100 $g/kg^{0,75}$ etwa in derselben Höhe wie im vorliegenden Versuch. Zudem müssen für eine sichere Defaunierung anscheinend auch die übrigen Randbedingungen (pelletierte Form, ein Kraftfutter vorwiegend aus Getreide, keine Aufteilung der Gabe), wie sie von der englischen Arbeitsgruppe um EADIE beschrieben worden sind, eingehalten werden. Auch aus der Untersuchung von CHRISTIANSEN u. a. (1964) ergibt sich zwingend, daß die Pelletierung die Defaunierungswirkung steigert.

Durch die in der vorliegenden Arbeit ausgeführten *in-vitro*-Experimente wurde versucht, den möglichen Ursachen eines Defaunierungseffektes der beschriebenen Kraftfuttermischung nachzugehen. Der Grund für die Wirkung der Gerste-Soja-Mischung auf die Protozoen dürfte in erster Linie im pH-absenkenden Effekt dieses stärkereichen Futters liegen. Es ist bekannt, daß Protozoen empfindlich gegen einen tiefen pH-Wert sind (PURSER und MOIR, 1959). Dies wurde in der vorliegenden Arbeit durch Säurezulagen *in vitro* demonstriert. *In vivo* dürfte bei der normalerweise üblichen Fütterungsweise der Säureabfluß aus dem Pansen bzw. die Resorption bei höheren pH-Werten hoch genug sein, um eine vollständige Defaunierung zu verhindern. Nach EADIE u. a. (1967) reicht es aber zur Defaunierung *in vivo* sogar aus, wenn der pH-Wert bis auf 5 fluktuiert. Aus dem Verlauf der Absenkung des pH-Wertes nach restriktiver Verabreichung des Kraftfutters (Tab. 2) wird zudem der anfänglich pH-stabilisierende Effekt der Protozoen offenbar. Dies ist möglicherweise eine der wichtigsten Aufgaben der Protozoen im Pansen bei Verfütterung stärkereicher Rationen (EADIE und MANN, 1970), da die Stärke von den Protozoen vor dem bakteriellen Zugriff weitgehend geschützt und nur langsam vergoren wird (COLEMAN, 1980). Außerdem scheinen sie eine höhere Aktivität im Abbau der bei hoher Stärkeaufnahme vermehrt entstehenden Milchsäure aufzuweisen als Bakterien (NEWBOLD u. a., 1985). Wird jedoch zuviel Stärke zugeführt, so ist die Kapazität der Protozoenpopulation erschöpft und die Bakterien produzieren große Mengen Säure aus Stärke (COLEMAN, 1979). Sinkt dann der pH-Wert unter 5, so fällt der Stabilisierungseffekt zusammen mit den Protozoen weg und es erfolgt ein zunächst ungebremster Abfall des pH-Werts, bis die Pansengärung zum Erliegen kommt. Es war daher in der vorliegenden Arbeit bei Färsen nicht möglich, eine Kraftfuttermenge zu bestimmen, bei der gerade eine Defaunierung erfolgt, der pH-Wert aber nicht unter 5 abfällt.

Die vorliegende Untersuchung gibt aber auch Hinweise dafür, daß die bei Pansenazidose in größeren Mengen gebildete Milchsäure noch eine zusätzliche Wirkung gegen Protozoen aufweist, die nicht durch den gesunkenen pH-Wert zu erklären ist. Für nicht identifizierte Defaunierungseffekte speziell der Gerste, wie sie von WHITELAW u. a. (1972) unterstellt wurden, ergaben sich in der vorliegenden Untersuchung keine Anhaltspunkte, da Weizen sogar schneller wirkte als Gerste. Eine etwas verzögerte Wirkung war dagegen bei Einsatz von Mais zu beobachten, was in einer stabileren Struktur der Stärkekörner im Vergleich zu Stärke aus Getreide begründet sein könnte (SUTTON, 1976). Je mehr Rohfaser die Ration enthält, umso geringer fällt die defaunierende Wirkung aus. Dies wird beim Einsatz von Hafer anstelle von Gerste, beim Vergleich von Kraftfutter I und II sowie beim Zusatz von Heu, Zellulose und Lignin deutlich. Wenig Bedeutung scheinen Pektine und Hemizellulosen zu haben. Bei den *in-vitro*-Versuchen konnte jedoch die meist eng mit dem Rohfasergehalt verknüpfte Strukturverbesserung nicht simuliert werden. Der dadurch möglicherweise erhöhte Fluß von Natriumbikarbonat in den Pansen dürfte jedoch keine bedeutende Änderung bringen, wie aus den *in-vitro*-Versuchen mit Puffersubstanzen abzuleiten ist.

Durch die starke Azidosegefahr ist Defaunierung mit Kraftfutter bei Färsen auch nach Gewöhnung an das Kraftfutter problematisch (vgl. auch EADIE u. a., 1970), wohingegen bei an eine sehr intensive Fütterung gewöhnten Bullen und Lämmern damit anscheinend problemlos ein protozoenfreier Zustand erreicht werden kann. Daraus ist zu schließen, daß diese Art der Defaunierung nur bei solchen Tieren gefahrlos möglich ist, die entweder sehr langsam an immer höhere Kraftfuttermengen gewöhnt werden bzw. diese bereits seit längerer Zeit erhalten (Kraftfuttermast), falls sie dann überhaupt noch eine Fauna besitzen. Die dabei über eine permanente latente Azidose hervorgerufene Verhornung des Pansenepithels dürfte der Verträglichkeit eher förderlich sein. Es ist aber mit einer großen Variation von Tier zu Tier bezüglich der ad-lib.-Aufnahme und der Reaktion auf das Kraftfutter zu rechnen (EADIE u. a., 1970).

4.2. Defaunierung mit Milch

Die ersten Versuche zur Defaunierung mit Milch wurden von EBERLEIN (1895) ausgeführt. Die Idee dazu ergab sich aus der Beobachtung, daß ausschließlich mit Milch gefütterte Jungtiere obligatorisch protozoenfrei sind. Eine 24stündige ad-lib.-Vorlage von Milch an ein 5 Wochen altes weibliches Ziegenlamm, das bereits eine Fauna aufwies, führte dann auch im Versuch von EBERLEIN (1895) zur Defaunierung. Bei einem 10 Wochen alten weiblichen Ziegenlamm mußte er drei Tage lang je 2×250 ml einflößen, um das Tier von Protozoen zu befreien. Die Befunde von EBERLEIN (1895) wurden von DOGIEL und WINOGRADOWA-FEDOROWA (1930) in Frage gestellt, da sie bei einer ausgewachsenen Ziege 6 Tage lang je einen Liter Milch verabreichen mußten, um eine Defaunierung zu bewirken. Diese Zeitspanne war sogar nur einen Tag kürzer, als es dauerte, das Tier durch Hungern zu defaunieren. GÜNTHER (1899) stellte überhaupt keine Wirkung von Milch gegen Protozoen fest, als er ein 5 Wochen altes männliches Ziegenlamm mit bereits entwickelter Fauna 11 Tage lang ausschließlich Milch ernährte. Für die fehlende Wirkung könnte hier jedoch ein noch vorhandener Schlundrinnenreflex verantwortlich gewesen sein (vgl. ØRSKOV und BENZIE, 1969). Der Panseninhalt war zu Ende des Versuchs von GÜNTHER (1899) jedenfalls nur schwach sauer. In einem neueren Experiment beschreiben KURIHARA u. a. (1978), daß Defaunierung von Schafen durch Magermilch (200 g/Tag) möglich sei. Dies wurde jedoch nur an einem Tier (42 kg) untersucht.

Die vorliegenden Versuche zeigen, daß durchaus von einem gewissen Effekt von Milch, insbesondere von Milchfett, gegen Protozoen ausgegangen werden kann, wenn auch vielleicht nicht mit der Deutlichkeit von Kraftfutter. Dies wurde *in vivo* (Tab. 6) und *in vitro* (Tab. 7) nachgewiesen. Aus Angaben zum Pansensaftvolumen von Lämmern (45 kg: 4,5–6 Liter; ORPIN und LETCHER, 1983/84) und Kühen (650 kg: 60–80 Liter; SNYDER u. a., 1984) kann abgeschätzt werden, daß die *in vivo* verabreichten Milchmengen einen Anteil zwischen 5 und 10 % am Pansensaft ausmachten, also eher die untere Grenze der *in-vitro*-Versuche repräsentierten.

Wie läßt sich der Defaunierungseffekt von Milch erklären? Es ist offensichtlich, daß man die Wirkung nicht von Beobachtungen an noch nicht ruminierenden Tieren ableiten kann, da bei diesen Tieren der pH-Wert im Pansen weit unter der für Protozoen kritischen Schwelle liegt. Andererseits fällt der pH-Wert in einem bereits ausgebildeten Pansen durch Nüchterung allein nicht mehr weit genug ab, sollte die Milch wegen des Schlundrinnenreflexes gar nicht in den Pansen gelangen. KURIHARA u. a. (1978) gehen sogar von einer Erhöhung des pH-Werts im Pansensaft als Ursache für die Wirkung von Magermilch gegen Protozoen aus, da er in ihrem Versuch auf 8 gestiegen war. Dafür gibt es in der vorliegenden Untersuchung keine Anhaltspunkte. Es wurde dagegen nachgewiesen, daß die Wirkung von Milch gegen Protozoen auf das enthaltene Fett zurückzuführen ist (Tabelle 7). In der Literatur finden sich Hinweise darauf, daß Öle,

z. B. aus Leinsaat und Kokosnuß, als Rationsbestandteile (5–7 %) die Fauna sehr deutlich vermindern (CZERKAWSKI u. a., 1975; IKWUEGBU und SUTTON, 1982; SUTTON u. a., 1983) und *in vitro* toxisch gegen Protozoen wirken (VAN NEVEL und DEMEYER, 1981). KAYOULI u. a. (1986) halten es deshalb für erfolgversprechend, längerkettige Fettsäuren zur Defaunierung einzusetzen. Die in der vorliegenden Untersuchung eingesetzten Fette zeigten keine Wirkung oder eine geringere Wirkung als Milchfett. Beim Sojaöl war die Verteilung nicht gewährleistet, die emulgierte Fettmischung „Micafett“ enthielt harte oder aufgehärtete Fette, wodurch möglicherweise die Wirkung gegen Protozoen verringert war. Milchfett weist dagegen 25–40 % ungesättigte Fettsäuren auf und hat damit einen Ölcharakter, besitzt aber im Gegensatz zu den meisten Ölen auch relativ hohe Anteile an kurzkettigen Fettsäuren (KIRCHGESSNER u. a., 1965). Die übrigen wichtigeren Milchbestandteile wie Laktose und verschiedene Milchproteinfraktionen in Kombination (Magermilch) oder einzeln (Kasein, Molke) erwiesen sich als praktisch unwirksam gegen Protozoen. Anhaltspunkte für eine Interaktionswirkung mit Fett sind nicht gegeben. Laktose (JOUANY und SENAUD, 1983) und Molkenpulver (GRUMMER u. a., 1983) beeinträchtigen auch in hohen Rationsanteilen die Fauna *in vivo* keineswegs.

Die praktische Anwendung der Defaunierung mit Milch scheint relativ problemlos zu sein, insbesondere auch was gesundheitliche Aspekte betrifft. Allerdings ist bei höherer Anflutung des sehr leicht abbaubaren Milchproteins die Gefahr einer Pansenfäule gegeben (Proteolyse durch Clostridien). Dies kann durch die Verwendung eiweißarmer bzw. fettreicher Milchprodukte (Sahne) umgangen werden. Die Toleranzgrenze des Wiederkäuers für Nahrungsfett (HAGEMEISTER und KAUFMANN, 1979) wird bei der Defaunierung mit Milch nicht erreicht, allerdings wird bei Defaunierung mit Sahne das Fett fast als alleinige Nahrungskomponente verabreicht, und nicht, wie üblich, als Mischungskomponente in Anteilen unter 10 %. Milch kann im Gegensatz zum Kraftfutter nicht über den Trog verabreicht werden, sondern muß über Flaschen eingegeben werden, weil sie von älteren Tieren in größeren Mengen nicht mehr freiwillig aufgenommen wird (vgl. EBERLEIN, 1895). Damit dürfte aber auch sichergestellt sein, daß der Schlundrinnenreflex nicht mehr ausgelöst wird (ØRSKOV und BENZIE, 1969).

Die Ergebnisse bei der nutritiven Defaunierung ergeben auch Anhaltspunkte dafür, wie ein einmal erreichter protozoenfreier Zustand ohne großen Aufwand (Isolierung, Desinfektion usw.) erhalten werden könnte. Die Fauna wird sich nämlich auch bei einer Neuinfektion kaum mehr in größerem Umfang etablieren können, wenn z. B. Öle in die Ration miteinbezogen werden. Dies hätte außer der Wirkung gegen Protozoen auch noch eine verbesserte Energieversorgung zur Folge, was für die Mast günstig zu bewerten ist. Andere Methoden zur kontinuierlichen Defaunierung mit Detergentien sind bisher gescheitert (BOODOO u. a., 1978) und zudem wieder mit den üblichen Nachteilen chemischer Methoden behaftet.

Zusammenfassung

In der vorliegenden Arbeit wurden zwei Möglichkeiten zur einfachen Defaunierung des Pansens mit Fütterungsmaßnahmen (nutritive Defaunierung) beim Wiederkäuer untersucht. Vorgehensweise und Wirksamkeit wurden dabei an Lämmern und Färsen erprobt. Als grundsätzlich geeignet erwiesen sich jeweils im Anschluß an eine kurzzeitige Nüchterung die ad-lib.-Verfütterung von pelletiertem Kraftfutter sowie der Einsatz von Milch (5–10 % des Pansensaftvolumens) und insbesondere von Milchfett (Sahne) zur Abtötung der Fauna. Defaunierung mit Kraftfutter war allerdings nur bei solchen Tieren gefahrlos möglich, die an eine sehr intensive Fütterung adaptiert waren.

In einer Reihe von *in-vitro*-Versuchen wurde den Wirkungsmechanismen der Methoden gegen die Protozoen nachgegangen. Hohe Mengen eines stärkereichen Kraftfutters wirkten vor allem aufgrund der pH-absenkenden Wirkung toxisch gegen Protozoen. Die entstehende Milchsäure verstärkte die Wirkung. Die defaunierende Wirkung des Kraftfutters wurde durch Zulage an Rohfaser (insbesondere Zellulose und Lignin) deutlich vermindert oder sogar unterbunden, wohingegen ein Pufferzusatz ohne Wirkung blieb. Die Defaunierung mit Milch wurde durch das enthaltene Milchfett bewirkt, während die übrigen quantitativen Milchinhaltsstoffe keinen Effekt zeigten.

Резюме

М. Крейцер и М. Кирхгесснер

Исследование по нутритивной дефаунизации рубца жвачных

В данной стате сообщают о двух методах простой дефаунизации рубца путём мероприятий при кормлении жвачных, т. е. с помощью нутритивной дефаунизации. Способ и действие проверялись в опытах на ягнятах и тёлках. В принципе благополучено для нарушения фауны было неперерывно после недлительной фазы натощака кормление вволю гранулированных концентратов, молока (5–10 % ёмкости рубцовой жидкости) и особенно молочного жира (сливки). Дефаунизация с помощью концентратов была только тогда безопасно возможной, если животные заранее адаптировались к такому очень интенсивному кормлению.

С помощью ряд опытов *in vitro* изучали механизм действия применяемых методов на простейшие. Высокие количества концентрата богатого крахмалом действовали токсически на простейшие из-за снижения pH. При этом образующаяся молочная кислота усиливалась это действие. Добавление клетчатки, в основном целлюлозы и лигнина, вело к значительному сокращению или даже утилизации дефаунизации впоследствии кормления концентратами. При добавке буфера наоборот никакого действия. Дефаунизация с помощью молока произошла из-за содержащего молочного жира, а все другие количественные ингредиенты молока не показали никакого эффекта.

Summary

M. Kreuzer and M. Kirchgessner

Investigations on the nutritive defaunation of the rumen of ruminants

Two promising methods to remove the ciliate protozoa of the stomach of ruminants by simple alterations in the feeding system were examined *in vivo* with lambs and heifers in the present investigation. The use of pelleted concentrates fed ad libitum and of milk, especially of milk fat (cream), turned out to be effective against protozoa when given after few hours of fasting. Milk led to the defaunation of a great proportion of the animals supplied all at once in an amount of 5–10 % of rumen fluid volume. With cream the amount could be lower according to the higher fat content. Defaunation with concentrate was found to be not dangerous only for animals adapted to intensive feeding sufficiently.

Additionally, a series of *in vitro* experiments were carried out to evaluate the reasons for the anti-protozoal effects of these methods. Concentrates rich in starch had toxic effects against protozoa, which mainly derived out of the depression in ruminal pH. The formed lactic acid had further effects irrespective of pH. The addition of crude fibre, especially of cellulose or lignin, reduced or prevented the anti-protozoal effects of concentrate fed ad lib. This was not so with the addition of buffers. With milk the included fat was shown to be responsible for the anti-protozoal effects, while the other main constituents of milk were of no importance.

Literaturverzeichnis

[1] BOODOO, A., B. HULMAN, T. R. PRESTON und R. A. LENG: Trop. Anim. Prod. **3**, 134 (1978)

[2] BURGGRAAF, W.: Thesis, Univ. New England, Armidale, Australia (1980) (zit. nach: BIRD, S. H. und R. A. LENG: Br. J. Nutrit. **52**, 607 (1984))

[3] CHRISTIANSEN, W. C., W. WOODS und W. BURROUGHS: J. Anim. Sci. **23**, 984 (1964)

[4] COLEMAN, G. S.: Trop. Anim. Prod. **4**, 199 (1979)

[5] COLEMAN, G. S.: Adv. Parasit. **18**, 121 (1980)

[6] CZERKAWSKI, J. W., W. W. CHRISTIE, GRACE BRECKENRIDGE und MARGARET L. HUNTER: Br. J. Nutrit. **34**, 25 (1975)

[7] DOGIEL, V. und T. WINOGRADOWA-FEDOROWA: Arch. Tierernähr. Tierzucht **3**, 172 (1930)

[8] EADIE, J. MARGARET und S. O. MANN: In: Proc. 3rd Int. Symp. Physiology of Digestion and Metabolism in the Ruminant (A. T. PHILLIPSON, ed.), Oriel Press, Newcastle upon Tyne, England, p. 335 ff (1970)

[9] EADIE, J. MARGARET und W. J. SHAND: Proc. Nutr. Soc. **40**, 113 A (1981)

[10] EADIE, J. MARGARET, P. N. HOBSON und S. O. MANN: Anim. Prod. **9**, 247 (1967)

[11] EADIE, J. MARGARET, J. HYLDGAARD-JENSEN, S. O. MANN, R. S. REID und F. G. WHITELAW: Br. J. Nutrit. **24**, 157 (1970)

[12] EBERLEIN, R.: Z. wiss. Zool. **59**, 233 (1895)

[13] GRUMMER, R. R., C. R. STAPLES und C. L. DAVIS: J. Dairy Sci. **66**, 1738 (1983)

[14] GÜNTHER, A.: Z. wiss. Zool. **65**, 529 (1899)

[15] HAGEMEISTER, H. und W. KAUFMANN: Übers. Tierernähr. **7**, 1 (1979)

[16] IKWUEGBU, O. A. und J. D. SUTTON: Br. J. Nutrit. **48**, 365 (1982)

[17] JOHNSON, R. R.: J. Anim. Sci. **43**, 184 (1976)

[18] JOUANY, J. P. und J. SENAUD: Ann. Biol. Anim. Bioch. Biophys. **19**, 619 (1979)

[19] JOUANY, J. P. und J. SENAUD: Reprod. Nutr. Develop. **23**, 607 (1983)

[20] KAYOULI, C., C. J. VAN NEVEL, R. DENDOOVEN und D. I. DEMEYER: Arch. Anim. Nutr. **36**, 827 (1986)

[21] KIRCHGESSNER, M., H. FRIESECKE und G. KOCH: Fütterung und Milchzusammensetzung. Bayerischer Landwirtschaftsverlag München (1965)

[22] KLOPFENSTEIN, T. J., D. B. PURSER und W. J. TYZNIK: J. Anim. Sci. **25**, 765 (1966)

[23] KREUZER, M.: J. Vet. Med. A **33**, 721 (1986)

[24] KREUZER, M. und M. KIRCHGESSNER: J. Anim. Physiol. Anim. Nutr. **56**, 217 (1986)

[25] KREUZER, M. und M. KIRCHGESSNER: J. Anim. Physiol. Anim. Nutr. Im Druck (1987)

[26] KREUZER, M., M. KIRCHGESSNER und H. L. MÜLLER: Anim. Feed Sci. Technol. **16**, 233 (1986)

[27] KURIHARA, Y., T. TAKECHI und F. SHIBATA: J. agric. Sci. **90**, 373 (1978)
[28] LEINMÜLLER, EDITH und K. H. MENKE: Übers. Tierernähr. **14**, 75 (1986)
[29] LOVELOCK, L. K. A., J. G. BUCHANAN-SMITH und C. W. FORSBERG: Canad. J. Anim. Sci. **62**, 299 (1982)
[30] MACKIE, R. I., FRANCES M. C. GILCHRIST, ANNA M. ROBBERTS, P. E. HANNAH und HELEN M. SCHWARTZ: J. agric. Sci. **90**, 241 (1978)
[31] MALES, J. R. und D. B. PURSER: Appl. Microbiol. **19**, 485 (1970)
[32] MENKE, K. H., L. RAAB, A. SALEWSKI. H. STEINGASS, D. FRITZ und W. SCHNEIDER: J. agric. Sci. **93**, 217 (1979)
[33] NEWBOLD, C. J., D. G. CHAMBERLAIN und A. G. WILLIAMS: Proc. Nutr. Soc. **44**, 85 A (1985)
[34] ORPIN, C. G.: J. Appl. Bacteriol. **43**, 309 (1977)
[35] ORPIN, C. G. und A. J. LETCHER: Anim. Feed Sci. Technol. **10**, 145 (1983/84)
[36] ØRSKOV, E. R. und D. BENZIE: Br. J. Nutrit. **23**, 415 (1969)
[37] PURSER, D. B. und R. J. MOIR: Aust. J. agric. Res. **10**, 555 (1959)
[38] SNYDER, T. J., L. D. MULLER, J. A. ROGERS und S. M. ABRAMS: J. Dairy Sci. **67**, 1953 (1984)
[39] SUTTON, J. D.: In: Principles of Cattle Production (SWAN, H. und W. H. BROSTER, eds). Butterworths, London, 121 (1976)
[40] SUTTON, J. D., R. KNIGHT, A. B. MCALLAN und R. H. SMITH: Br. J. Nutrit. **49**, 419 (1983)
[41] TAKAHASHI, F. und M. KAMETAKA: Jap. J. Zootech. Sci. **47**, 192 (1976)
[42] VAN NEVEL, C. J. und D. I. DEMEYER: Arch. Tierernähr. **31**, 141 (1981)
[43] VEIRA, D. M.: J. Anim. Sci. **63**, 1547 (1986)
[44] WHITELAW, F. G., J. MARGARET EADIE, S. O. MANN und R. S. REID: Br. J. Nutrit. **27**, 425 (1972)
[45] WHITELAW, F. G., J. MARGARET EADIE, L. A. BRUCE und W. J. SHAND: Br. J. Nutrit. **52**, 261 (1984)

Eingegangen: 26. Januar 1987

Anschrift der Autoren:
Prof. Dr. M. KIRCHGESSNER und Dr. M. KREUZER, Institut für Ernährungsphysiologie der Technischen Universität München
D - 8050 Freising-Weihenstephan
BRD

Buchbesprechung

Futterproduktion. Verfasser: W. BREUNIG, B. MÄRTIN und E. WOHJAHN. Berlin, VEB Deutscher Landwirtschaftsverlag 1986. 388 Seiten, DDR 31,– M

Aufgaben und praktische Maßnahmen bei der Intensivierung der Produktion und Bereitstellung von Grobfutter sind Gegenstand des unter Federführung von BREUNIG (Berlin), MÄRTIN (Halle) und WOJAHN (Paulinenaue) verfaßten Hochschullehrbuches „Futterproduktion". Das in der DDR erstmalig erschienene Werk behandelt in komplexer Weise den Anbau, die Ernte, Konservierung und Lagerung von Grobfutter. Die Strohaufbereitung zu Futterzwecken sowie die Konservierung von Futterhackfrüchten werden ebenfalls dargelegt. Es verdient besondere Anerkennung, daß dem Lehrbuch eine betont futterwirtschaftliche Betrachtungsweise zugrunde liegt. So werden eine Vielzahl von Maßnahmen zur intensiven Grobfutterproduktion aus den Bedarfsforderungen der Tierproduktion abgeleitet. Als praktische Lösungswege zur Aufnahme und Verwertung großer Energie- und Nährstoffanteile aus dem Grobfutter nennen die Autoren vor allem die Bereitstellung von mehr Frischfutter einschl. der Nutzung der Intensivweide, die entschiedene Qualitätsverbesserung bei den Konservaten sowie eine exaktere Erfassung und Bewertung der Grobfuttermengen und -qualitäten in jeder Kooperation.

Die Darstellung naturwissenschaftlicher, agronomischer sowie technisch-technologischer Grundlagen, Zusammenhänge und Maßnahmen wird vorwiegend aus der Sicht ihrer volks- und betriebswirtschaftlichen Effektivität vorgenommen. Ein gesonderter Abschnitt zur Ökonomik der Futterproduktion vervollständigt die Gesamtaussage des Buches ebenso wie der interessante Überblick über Stand und Entwicklungsrichtungen der Futterproduktion in einigen Hauptregionen der Welt, an dem auch Wissenschaftler aus der UdSSR mitwirkten.

Erstmalig in der DDR wird in dem vorliegenden Hochschullehrbuch die Gesamtheit der Grobfutterproduktion abgehandelt; nach dem Ackerfutter mit seinen zahlreichen Haupt- und Zwischenfruchtpflanzen und deren Gemengen findet das Grasland eine sehr umfangreiche Berücksichtigung. Die praktische Relevanz des Buches wird erhöht durch eine starke Orientierung auf die unterschiedlichen natürlichen und ökonomischen Standortbedingungen.

Insgesamt spricht das Hochschullehrbuch durch Aufbau, Gestaltung und Inhalt die in Lehre, Forschung, Studium und sozialistischer Praxis tätigen Pflanzen- und Tierproduzenten gleichermaßen an.

E. KABIS

Arch. Anim. Nutr., Berlin 37 (1987) 6, 505–520

Sektion Tierproduktion und Veterinärmedizin der Karl-Marx-Universität Leipzig,
Wissenschaftsbereich Tierernährungschemie
(Leiter: Prof. Dr. sc. agr. A. HENNIG)

K. GRUHN und G. JAHREIS

Dynamik des Aminosäuren- und Proteinstoffwechsels der Legehennen nach Applikation von ^{15}N-markiertem Weizenprotein

2. *Mitteilung*

^{15}N-Exkretion mit dem Stickstoff und den basischen Aminosäuren des Kotes

1. Einleitung

^{15}N-markierte Futtermittel erlauben nach Erreichung des ^{15}N-Plateaus im Kot die Einschätzung des resorbierten ^{15}N-Anteiles des Futters, da eine Falsifizierung durch ^{15}N-Substanzen endogenen Ursprungs noch gering ist. HENNIG und GRUHN (1978) konnten an kolostomierten Legehennen eine mittlere scheinbare Verdaulichkeit des Stickstoffes mit natürlicher Häufigkeit der Ration von 80,2 % und für die Verdaulichkeit des Weizen-^{15}N eine signifikant höhere von 86,0 % nachweisen. In dieser Versuchsreihe war es möglich, nach dem Absetzen des markierten Weizens die Hennen zu vier verschiedenen Zeitpunkten zu schlachten. Dadurch konnte im Vergleich zu früheren Versuchen mit ^{15}N′-Kasein (HENNIG u. a., 1975) und ^{15}N′-Weizen (HENNIG und GRUHN, 1978) eine detailliertere Aussage zur Exkretion von Stickstoff und Aminosäuren mit dem Kot sowie der Verdaulichkeit des Rohproteins und der Resorption von Aminosäuren getroffen werden.

2. Methodik

2.1. Hennen und deren Haltung

Für den Versuch standen 12 kolostomierte Leghorn zur Verfügung, die 4 Tage mit der Ration ^{15}N-markierten Weizen erhielten. 12 h, 36 h, 60 h und 108 h nach der letzten ^{15}N-Gabe wurden jeweils drei Tiere geschlachtet. Während der Versuchsdurchführung befanden sich die Hennen in der ersten Hälfte der Legetätigkeit. Die Haltung der Tiere erfolgte in Einzelkäfigen mit einer Grundfläche von 50 × 50 cm und Trennwänden aus Glas. Die Futternäpfe und Tränkbehälter als auch die austauschbaren Kotschieber bestanden aus Polyvinylchlorid. Der auf 20 °C temperierte Raum war von 6.00 ... 20.00 Uhr beleuchtet. Den Tieren stand Tränkwasser ad libitum zur Verfügung.

2.2. Futter und Fütterung

Die Mehrkomponentenration wurde zwecks quantitativer Futteraufnahme pelletiert. Der in der viertägigen Hauptperiode verfütterte markierte Weizen wies einen ^{15}N-Überschuß (^{15}N′) von 14,37 Atom-% auf. Die Markierung der basischen Aminosäuren betrug für Lysin 13,58 Atom-% $^{15}N'$, für Histidin 14,38 Atom-% $^{15}N'$ und für Arginin 13,63 Atom-% $^{15}N'$. Einzelheiten der Zusammensetzung der Ration und der Fütterung wurden von HENNIG u. a. (1987) mitgeteilt.

2.3. Analysenverfahren

Der Kot wurde von jeder Henne täglich viermal genommen und zur Sammelprobe vereinigt. In den Futtermitteln erfolgte die Bestimmung der Rohnährstoffe nach TGL 80-21 875. Die Garnitur der basischen Aminosäuren wurde in den einzelnen Futter- und Kotproben ermittelt. Außerdem erfolgte nach der von KIRCHNER und GRUHN (1985) mitgeteilten Prozedur die Fällung des Kotproteins mit Trichloressigsäure (TCE) und die Bestimmung des Stickstoffes sowohl im Kot als auch in der TCE-löslichen Fraktion. Die Ermittlung des schweren Stickstoffes erfolgte emissionsspektrometrisch, wobei die basischen Aminosäuren vorher am Präparativzusatz des Aminosäurenanalysators Unichrom getrennt wurden.

3. Ergebnisse und Diskussion

3.1. Exkretion an Gesamt-N und -$^{15}N'$

Bei einer täglichen Gesamt-N-Aufnahme von 3020 mg schwankte die mittlere tägliche N-Exkretion mit dem Kot zwischen 440 mg (Henne 9) und 636 mg (Henne 2). Im Mittel aller Hennen und Tage wurden 512 mg exkretiert (Abb. 1). Durch die hohe

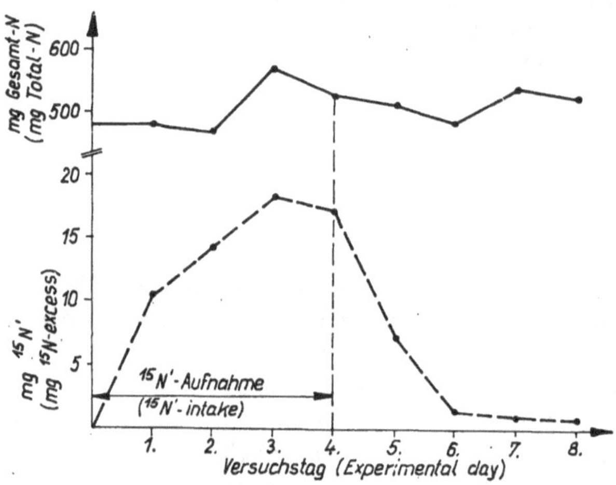

Abb. 1 (Fig. 1). Mittlere Exkretion an Gesamt-N und $^{15}N'$ mit dem Kot je Tier und Tag (Mean excretion of the total-N and $^{15}N'$ via faeces per animal and day).

Tierzahl konnte im Vergleich zu einem in der Anlage ähnlichen, von HENNIG und GRUHN (1978) durchgeführten Versuch mit nur drei Hennen eine fast ideale Kurve für den Verlauf der $^{15}N'$-Exkretion gefunden werden (Abb. 1). Bereits am Ende des 5. Versuchstages – einem Tag nach dem Absetzen des markierten Futters – war die Exkretion von unverdautem und resekretiertem $^{15}N'$ zu 94 % annähernd abgeschlossen, bei Unterstellung, daß die $^{15}N'$-Ausscheidung am letzten Versuchstag = 100 % beträgt (Tab. 1). Auf die letzten drei Versuchstage entfallen nur 6 % der Gesamtaus-

Tabelle 1 (Table 1)
Mittlere kumulative $^{15}N'$-Aufnahme und $^{15}N'$-Exkretion je Henne und Tag
(Mean cumulative $^{15}N'$-intake and $^{15}N'$-excretion per hen and day)

Versuchstag (Experimental day)	Hennenzahl (Number of hens)	$^{15}N'$-Aufnahme ($^{15}N'$-intake)* mg	mittlere $^{15}N'$-Exkretion (Mean mg	$^{15}N'$-excretion) relative %
1.	12	155	10,6	
2.	12	270	25,0	
3.	12	405	43,2	
4.	12	540	60,6	84
5.	9		67,9	94
6.	6		69,6	96
7.	3		70,9	98
8.	3		72,2	100

* ^{15}N-excess ($^{15}N'$)

scheidung. Die $^{15}N'$-Exkretion vom 6. bis 8. Versuchstag mit dem Kot beruht auf der endogenen Sekretion von $^{15}N'$ in das Darmlumen. Die endogene Sekretion erfolgt bereits im oberen Teil des Verdauungstraktes in Form von Speichel, ösophagealen Sekreten und Magensaft. Für die N-Anreicherung im Dünndarmlumen sind neben Pankreasenzymen (Bergner u. a., 1976; Figarella, 1973), desquaminierenden Mukosazellen und Mukoproteinen (Munro, 1964) auch Plasmaproteine (Armstrong u. a., 1960; Campbell u. a., 1961; Glass und Ishimori, 1961) sowie freie Aminosäuren (Nasset and Ju, 1961) verantwortlich.

Bird (1968) konnte bei Küken im Dünndarminhalt die vierfache Menge an endogenem Protein im Verhältnis zum exogenen ermitteln, während Crompton und Nesheim (1969) bei Enten nur die Hälfte des im Dünndarmlumen befindlichen Proteins als endogenes annahmen. Die genaue Ermittlung des endogenen Anteils ist methodisch sehr schwierig.

3.2. Scheinbare Verdaulichkeit von ^{14}N und $15N'$

Die Auswertung der Versuchsergebnisse wurde für die einzelnen Hennen und die einzelnen Versuchstage durchgeführt. In Tabelle 2 werden die kumulative Aufnahme und Exkretion mit dem Kot an ^{14}N und $^{15}N'$ sowie die scheinbare Verdaulichkeit für die einzelnen Versuchstiere innerhalb des Versuchszeitraumes mitgeteilt.

Die scheinbare Verdaulichkeit des ^{14}N der Ration beträgt im Mittel 82,8 % ± 1,9 % und die scheinbare Verdaulichkeit des $^{15}N'$ vom Weizen 87,5 % ± 1,9 % (Tab. 2). Entsprechend den methodischen Anforderungen für die Durchführung von Verdauungsversuchen beim Geflügel (Wiesemüller, 1983) ist die Streuung der scheinbaren Verdaulichkeit des ^{14}N und $^{15}N'$ zwischen den einzelnen Versuchstieren mit <2 Verdaulichkeitseinheiten als gut einzuschätzen. Für die Differenzen zwischen der scheinbaren Verdaulichkeit des ^{14}N und $^{15}N'$ konnten für die jeweiligen Dreiergruppen nach viertägiger Versuchszeit 5,9 Verdaulichkeitseinheiten, nach fünf Tagen 4,9, nach sechs Tagen 3,9 und nach acht Tagen ebenfalls 3,9 Einheiten ermittelt werden (Tab. 2).

Diese Verminderung der Differenz in Abhängigkeit von der Zeit nach der letzten ^{15}N-Fütterung resultiert aus der Exkretion von $^{15}N'$ endogenen Ursprungs und führt somit zu einer falsifizierten Einschätzung der scheinbaren Verdaulichkeit. Aus diesem Grunde sollte für die Ermittlung der scheinbaren Verdaulichkeit des Weizen-$^{15}N'$ der Wert vom 3. und 4. Versuchstag der $^{15}N'$-Fütterung zugrunde gelegt werden. An den beiden

Tabelle 2 (Table 2)

Kumulative Aufnahme und Exkretion mit dem Kot an ^{14}N und $^{15}N'$ sowie die scheinbare Verdaulichkeit für die einzelnen Versuchstiere

(Cumulative intake and excretion of ^{14}N and $^{15}N'$ in faeces and the apparent digestibility for individual animals)

Hennen-Nr. (Number of hen)	Versuchstage (Experimental days)	^{14}N-Aufnahme (^{14}N-intake) mg	^{14}N-Exkretion (^{14}N-Excretion) mg	^{14}N-Verdaulichkeit (^{14}N-Digestibility) %	$^{15}N'$-Aufnahme ($^{15}N'$-Intake) mg	$^{15}N'$-Exkretion ($^{15}N'$-Excretion) mg	$^{15}N'$-Verdaulichkeit ($^{15}N'$-Digestibility) %
1	4	11540	1984	82,8	540	61,4	88,6
2	4	11540	2463	78,7	540	81,0	85,0
3	4	11540	1845	84,0	540	57,1	89,4
4	5	14560	2535	82,6	540	66,8	87,6
5	5	14560	2726	81,3	540	77,2	85,7
6	5	14560	2222	84,7	540	52,8	90,2
7	6	17580	2917	83,4	540	66,9	87,6
8	6	17580	2825	83,9	540	67,0	87,6
9	6	17580	2580	85,3	540	59,2	89,0
10	8	23620	4668	80,2	540	88,8	83,6
11	8	23620	4088	82,7	540	68,9	87,2
12	8	23620	3688	84,4	540	64,0	88,2

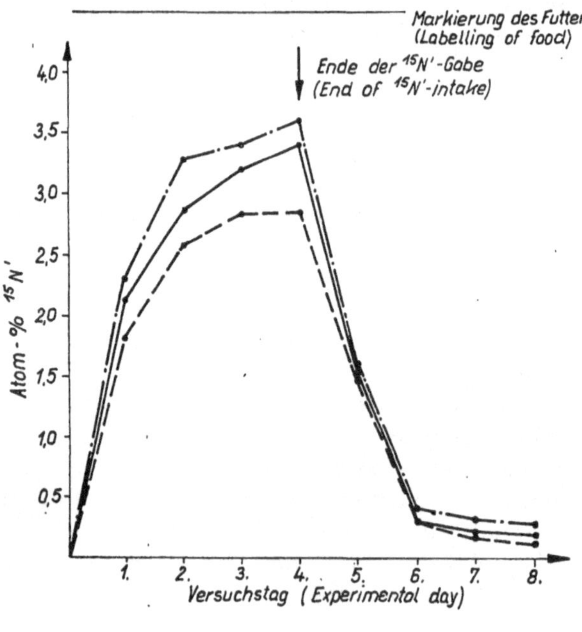

Abb. 2 (Fig. 2). Atom-% $^{15}N'$ des gesamten Kotes und der Kotfraktionen in Abhängigkeit von der Versuchszeit (Atom-% of $^{15}N'$ of total faeces and faecal fractions dependent on trial length). ——— Gesamt-$^{15}N'$ (Total-$^{15}N'$) —·—· TCE-fällbarer $^{15}N'$ (TCA-precipitable $^{15}N'$) – – – TCE-löslicher $^{15}N'$ (TCA-soluble $^{15}N'$).

Tagen wird ein Plateau (steady state) in der ^{15}N-Häufigkeit erreicht (Abb. 2). Danach beträgt die scheinbare Verdaulichkeit des ^{15}N' vom Weizen 89,1 %, und zu der des ^{14}N mit 82,8 % besteht somit eine Differenz von sechs Verdaulichkeitseinheiten.

Von HENNIG und GRUHN (1978) konnte bei vergleichbarer Rationsgestaltung ebenfalls eine um 5,5 Einheiten bessere scheinbare Verdaulichkeit des Weizenproteins nachgewiesen werden.

Die Aufschlüsselung der ^{15}N'-Exkretion auf die Versuchstage ergibt eine vorgetäuschte hohe scheinbare Verdaulichkeit am 1. und 2. Versuchstag durch die Verweildauer im Gastrointestinaltrakt, worauf schon von HENNIG u. a. (1975) hingewiesen wurde. Bereits einen Tag nach Absetzen des markierten Weizens (5. Versuchstag) wird für die scheinbare Verdaulichkeit ein Mittelwert von 87,4 % errechnet und damit genau der Wert, der dem Mittel aller Hennen entspricht (Tab. 2).

Dieses Resultat spricht für die schnelle Passage des Futters bei Legehennen (HOFFMANN u. a. 1972).

3.3. TCE-fällbare und -lösliche N-Fraktion im Kot

Der Atom-% ^{15}N' der TCE-fällbaren N-Fraktion ist bereits nach dem ersten ^{15}N'-Applikationstag höher als in der Nichtprotein-N-Fraktion; er beträgt im Mittel 2,40 Atom-% ^{15}N' und in der NPN-Fraktion 1,87 Atom-% ^{15}N'. Die Unterschiede bleiben während der ^{15}N'-Gabe annähernd gleich. Die Markierung erreichte mit der letzten ^{15}N'-Applikation die höchsten Werte (Abb. 2); der mittlere ^{15}N' der Eiweißfraktion beträgt 3,48 Atom-% ^{15}N' und der der TCE-löslichen N-Fraktion 2,93 Atom-% ^{15}N'. Der Maximalwert des Gesamt-^{15}N' von 3,30 Atom-% entspricht zu 74 % der Markierungshöhe des Futtereiweißes. Am letzten Versuchstag ist die Markierung des Stickstoffes beider Fraktionen, der ausschließlich endogenen Ursprungs ist, etwa gleich (Abb. 2). Die Differenz der Markierungshöhe vom TCE-löslichen N zum Gesamt-N im Kot beträgt etwa das Doppelte im Vergleich zur Differenz des TCE-fällbaren N zum Gesamt-N. Die Unterschiede im Atom-% ^{15}N' ergeben sich aus dem Mengenverhältnis TCE-löslicher N zu fällbarem von 1 : 2 (Tab. 4). Hohe Werte im TCE-löslichen N

Tabelle 3 (Table 3)
Mittlerer Gehalt des Kotes an gesamtem und TCE-löslichem Stickstoff mit natürlicher isotoper Häufigkeit pro Tier und Tag
(Mean content of faeces of the total and TCA-soluble nitrogen with natural isotopic frequency per animal and day)

Versuchstag (Experimental day)	gesamter ^{14}N (total ^{14}N) mg	s±	TCE-löslicher ^{14}N (TCA-soluble ^{14}N) mg	s±	relativ % (relative %) $\bar{x}$	s±
1.	465	74	159	27	34,2	2,6
2.	460	74	157	30	34,1	3,2
3.	555	94	181	31	32,7	2,5
4.	508	113	164	28	32,7	3,0
5.	510	50	170	14	33,5	1,9
6.	480	90	164	32	34,2	2,1
7.	543	88	179	15	33,4	2,9
8.	523	114	175	48	33,3	2,5

werden durch niedrige in der TCE-fällbaren N-Fraktion kompensiert und umgekehrt (HENNIG und GRUHN, 1978).

Wir haben den TCE-löslichen Stickstoff mit natürlicher isotoper Häufigkeit (^{14}N) zum gesamten ^{14}N relativiert und zu dem mit schwerem Stickstoff verglichen (Tab. 3).

Bemerkenswerterweise beträgt der TCE-lösliche ^{14}N-Anteil etwa ein Drittel an dem gesamten ^{14}N (Tab. 3). Dieses Verhältnis kann als typisch für Legehennenkot angesehen werden. JAHREIS und GRUHN (1979) konnten bei Broilerzuchthennen die gleichen Relationen ermitteln. Enthält die Ration dagegen hochverdauliche Eiweißkomponenten, wie z. B. Kasein, kann der TCE-lösliche N-Anteil im Kot-N der Henne auf über 50 % ansteigen (HENNIG u. a., 1975). Während beim nichtmarkierten Rationsstickstoff der Nichtprotein-N-Anteil ein Drittel ausmachte, beträgt der nicht fällbare $^{15}N'$-Anteil vom gesamten Kot-$^{15}N'$ im Mittel nicht über 30 %, wobei der lösliche Anteil am zweiten Tag nach dem Absetzen auf 32,6 % steigt (Tab. 4) und mit

Tabelle 4 (Table 4)
Mittlerer Gehalt an gesamtem und TCE-löslichem schweren Stickstoff pro Tier und Tag
(Mean content of total and TCA-soluble heavy nitrogen per animal and day)

Versuchs-tag (Experimental day)	gesamter $^{15}N'$ mg (total $^{15}N'$ mg) $\bar{x}$	s ±	TCE-löslicher $^{15}N'$ mg (TCA-soluble $^{15}N'$ mg) $\bar{x}$	s ±	relativ % (relative %) $\bar{x}$	s ±
1.	10,57	2,63	3,04	0,67	29,0	3,0
2.	14,41	2,77	4,19	0,89	29,2	3,2
3.	18,27	3,38	5,07	1,12	27,7	3,2
4.	17,39	5,30	4,97	1,53	28,8	3,4
5.	7,29	1,86	2,05	0,47	28,3	1,7
6.	1,62	0,42	0,53	0,16	32,6	3,2
7.	1,35	0,33	0,39	0,10	28,1	4,7
8.	1,34	0,27	0,33	0,08	24,8	5,7

dem vermehrten Ausschütten von löslichen markierten N-Verbindungen in das Darmlumen im Zusammenhang stehen dürfte. Am Versuchsende fällt der $^{15}N'$-Anteil auf 24,8 % ab. Die futterbürtigen, in der TCE-löslichen Fraktion befindlichen freien Aminosäuren und auch weitere NPN-Verbindungen dürften fast vollständig resorbiert werden, so daß die TCE-löslichen N-Verbindungen im wesentlichen endogener Herkunft sind bzw. durch bakterielle Proteolyse des unverdauten Proteins im Enddarm entstehen (PAYNE u. a., 1968; CROMPTON und NESHEIM, 1969).

3.4. Basische Aminosäuren

3.4.1. Aminosäurengehalt im Rohprotein und Protein des Kotes

Die Bestimmung der basischen Aminosäuren erfolgte sowohl nach Hydrolyse des Kotes als auch in der Fraktion des TCE-fällbaren Proteins. Die Werte an Aminosäuren wurden auf das Roh- bzw. Reinprotein bezogen und der Mittelwert wurde für jede Henne nachgewiesen (Tab. 5, 6).

Tabelle 5 (Table 5)
Mittlerer Gehalt an basischen Aminosäuren im Rohprotein des Kotes in Prozent
(Mean content of basic amino acids in crude protein of faeces in %)

Hennen-Nr. (Number of hen)	Lysin (Lysine) $\bar{x}$	s±	Histidin (Histidine) $\bar{x}$	s±	Arginin (Arginine) $\bar{x}$	s±
1	4,79	0,36	2,29	0,34	3,73	0,24
2	6,09	0,52	2,30	0,56	3,72	0,43
3	5,24	0,39	2,32	0,31	3,66	0,26
4	5,37	0,41	2,50	0,17	3,77	0,23
5	4,65	0,40	2,18	0,09	3,72	0,24
6	5,37	0,39	2,12	0,19	3,48	0,32
7	4,95	0,40	2,24	0,42	3,99	0,22
8	5,06	0,35	2,19	0,43	3,68	0,58
9	5,11	0,33	2,20	0,25	3,63	0,32
10	6,43	0,42	2,52	0,36	3,64	0,19
11	5,86	0,98	2,49	0,37	3,84	0,55
12	5,74	0,31	2,19	0,26	3,39	0,55

Tabelle 6 (Table 6)
Mittlerer Gehalt an basischen Aminosäuren im Reinprotein des Kotes in Prozent
(Mean content of basic amino acids in protein of faeces in %)

Hennen-Nr. (Number of hen)	Lysin (Lysine) $\bar{x}$	s±	Histidin (Histidine) $\bar{x}$	s±	Arginin (Arginine) $\bar{x}$	s±
1	5,72	0,34	2,31	0,25	4,26	0,41
2	6,50	0,69	2,77	0,35	4,50	0,75
3	5,51	0,69	2,42	0,29	4,31	0,51
4	5,03	0,83	2,24	0,17	4,18	0,62
5	4,76	0,44	2,04	0,13	4,11	0,38
6	4,58	0,39	1,85	0,15	3,26	0,19
7	5,69	0,37	2,44	0,24	4,39	0,43
8	5,24	0,41	2,42	0,35	3,93	0,47
9	5,33	0,23	2,15	0,14	4,24	0,40
10	5,67	0,42	2,53	0,28	4,19	0,67
11	5,55	0,56	2,27	0,14	3,78	0,21
12	5,55	0,49	2,36	0,29	3,73	0,36

Demnach liegen die Lysinwerte des Rohproteins der Hennen 2 und 10 über 6 % und die von Henne 5 und 7 unter 5 % (Tab. 5). Der Histidin- und Argininggehalt des Rohproteins ist zwischen den Hennen recht gut ausgeglichen und liegt zwischen 2,1 ... 2,5 % bzw. 3,4 ... 4,0 %. Ein Vergleich des Lysingehaltes in Prozent der gesamten N-Verbindungen (Tab. 5) und des echten Eiweißes (Tab. 6) zeigt, daß bei der Mehrheit der Tiere der Gehalt im Reineiweiß höher liegt, bei Arginin trifft es sogar für 10 Hennen zu. Dieser Vergleich weist auf eine Ausschüttung von Eiweißverbindungen endogener Herkunft in das Darmlumen hin, die nicht gespalten worden sind. Trotz des hohen Lysingehaltes im Rohprotein des Futters von 4,70 % liegt der mittlere Lysingehalt des Kotes der 12 Tiere mit 5,45 ± 0,71 g je 100 g Rohprotein um 16 % höher. Im Gegensatz dazu ist der Histidingehalt mit 2,32 ± 0,33 g je 100 g Kotroheiweiß um 18 % und der Arginingehalt mit 3,68 ± 0,39 g um 38 % niedriger als der des Futterrohproteins. Ähnliche Relationen wurden für die basischen Aminosäuren von HENNIG und GRUHN (1978) bei der Verfütterung von Weizenrationen an Legehennen ermittelt. Dieser Befund der Nichtübereinstimmung der Kot- und Futteraminosäurendaten ist auf die aktive Rolle des Darmes im Aminosäurenstoffwechsel zurückzuführen. Wie GRUHN (1974) sowie GRUHN und JAHREIS (1974) in weiteren Versuchen mit Geflügel nachweisen konnten, wird die Aminosäurengarnitur der Digesta im wesentlichen dem Pool des Körpers angeglichen, so daß auch bei extremer Futterproteinzusammensetzung kaum ein Einfluß auf den Aminosäurengehalt des Kotproteins nachweisbar ist. Diese Gesetzmäßigkeit konnten ZIMMER u. a. (1975) mit radioaktiv markierten Aminosäuren an Ratten bestätigen.

3.4.2. Basische Aminosäuren in der TCE-fällbaren $^{15}N'$-Fraktion

Die TCE-fällbare ^{15}'-Menge aus Lysin, Histidin und Arginin wurde zum entsprechenden gesamten Aminosäuren-$^{15}N'$ relativiert (Tab. 7).

Tabelle 7 (Table 7)
Mittlerer Anteil der TCE-fällbaren Aminosäure-$^{15}N'$-Fraktion an der entsprechenden gesamten Aminosäure-$^{15}N'$-Menge in Prozent
(Mean percentage of the TCA-precipitable amino acid-$^{15}N'$-fraction of the adequate total amino acid-$^{15}N'$-amount)

Versuchstag (Experimental day)	Lysin (Lysine) x̄	s±	Histidin (Histidine) x̄	s±	Arginin (Arginine) x̄	s±
1.	69,1	13,6	76,7	12,9	69,4	8,3
2.	71,9	8,1	71,4	13,5	74,4	14,0
3.	76,3	12,0	72,3	13,2	72,0	15,8
4.	70,6	7,0	73,6	12,0	68,3	12,6
5.	73,3	7,2	78,8	9,8	74,0	14,1
6.	66,7	13,1	81,3	5,1	83,4	6,6
7.	65,4	6,6	81,5	6,3	60,6	7,9
8.	63,1	4,3	70,5	15,4	63,2	12,6

Es konnten über das gewogene Mittel für Lysin-$^{15}N'$ 70,9 %, mit TCE gefällt, nachgewiesen werden. Die entsprechenden Mittelwerte für Histidin und Arginin betragen 73,7 % bzw. 70,3 %. Demnach liegen die TCE-löslichen $^{15}N'$-Anteile mit 29,1 % für Lysin bzw. mit 29,7 % für Arginin in der gleichen Größenordnung wie der TCE-lösliche $^{15}N'$-Anteil am gesamten $^{15}N'$ des Kotes (Tab. 4). Der lösliche $^{15}N'$-Anteil des Histidins mit 26,3 % am gesamten Histidin-$^{15}N'$ des Kotes liegt somit am niedrigsten von den geprüften Komponenten.

3.4.3. Atom-% $^{15}N'$ der basischen Aminosäuren

Die Markierung des Stickstoffes der basischen Aminosäuren steigt mit dem Beginn der $^{15}N'$-Applikation ebenso steil an (Abb. 3) wie die des gesamten Stickstoffes des Kotes (Abb. 2).

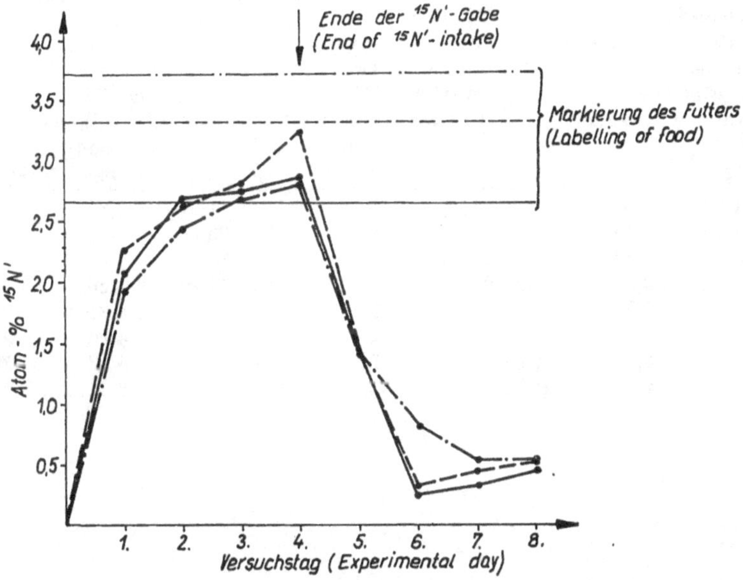

Abb. 3 (Fig. 3). Mittlerer Atom-% $^{15}N'$ von Lysin-N, Histidin-N und Arginin-N des Kotes im Vergleich zum Futter (Mean atom-% of $^{15}N'$ of lysine-N, histidine-N and arginine-N of faeces compared to rations). ——— Lysin (Lysine) —·— Histidin (Histidine) – – – Arginin (Arginine).

Am zweiten Tag der $^{15}N'$-Applikation entspricht der Atom-% $^{15}N'$ des Lysins dem des Futters und liegt am letzten Tag der $^{15}N'$-Gabe mit 3,0 Atom-% $^{15}N'$ etwas höher als der des Lysins der Futterration. Für die höhere Markierung des exkretierten Lysins (Abb. 3) ist der bereits erwähnte hohe Anteil dieser Aminosäure am Kotrohprotein (Tab. 5) bzw. Reinprotein (Tab. 6), der endogen bedingt ist, anzusehen. Von den basischen Aminosäuren liegt zwar die Markierung des Arginin-$^{15}N'$ am letzten Tag der $^{15}N'$-Applikation am höchsten, erreicht jedoch nicht ganz die Argininmarkierung von 3,36 Atom-% $^{15}N'$ des Futters (Abb. 3). Der Atom-% $^{15}N'$ des Kothistidins liegt mit 2,85 am letzten Tag der $^{15}N'$-Verabreichung nicht ganz so hoch wie der von Lysin und beträgt 76 % der Markierung des Histidins aus dem Futter, etwa die gleichen Relationen konnten für die Markierung des Kot-N (Abb. 2) im Vergleich zur Markierung des Futter-N von 4,47 Atom-% $^{15}N'$ nachgewiesen werden.

3.4.4. Exkretion des $^{15}N'$ mit den basischen Aminosäuren

Am fünften Versuchstag – einem Tag nach der letzten $^{15}N'$-Gabe – waren relativ zur im Versuchszeitraum exkretierten Aminosäuren-$^{15}N'$-Menge bei allen drei basischen Aminosäuren über 90 % im Kot ausgeschieden, wobei die kumulative Ausscheidung am letzten Versuchstag=100 % gesetzt wurde (Tab. 8).

Tabelle 8 (Table 8)

Mittlere kumulative Aufnahme und Exkretion je Henne und Tag von Lysin-$^{15}N'$, Histidin-$^{15}N'$ und Arginin-$^{15}N'$

(Mean cumulative intake and excretion of lysine-$^{15}N'$, histidine-$^{15}N'$ and arginine-$^{15}N'$ per animal and day)

Versuchs-tag (Experimental day)	Tierzahl (Number of animals)	Lysin-$^{15}N'$ Aufnahme (Lysine $^{15}N'$) (Intake)	Exkretion (Excretion)		Histidin-$^{15}N'$ Aufnahme (Histidine $^{15}N'$) (Intake)	Exkretion (Excretion)		Arginin-$^{15}N'$ Aufnahme (Arginine $^{15}N'$) (Intake)	Exkretion (Excretion)	
		mg	mg	%	mg	mg	%	mg	mg	%
1.	12	4,52	0,60		5,37	0,36		11,97	0,82	
2.	12	9,05	1,43		10,75	0,83		23,95	1,74	
3.	12	13,58	2,49		16,12	1,45		35,92	2,95	
4.	12	18,10	3,50	80	21,50	2,06	80	47,90	4,26	80
5.	9		3,99	92		2,35	91		4,84	91
6.	6		4,09	94		2,40	93		4,96	93
7.	3		4,21	97		2,50	97		5,13	97
8.	3		4,36	100		2,59	100		5,31	100

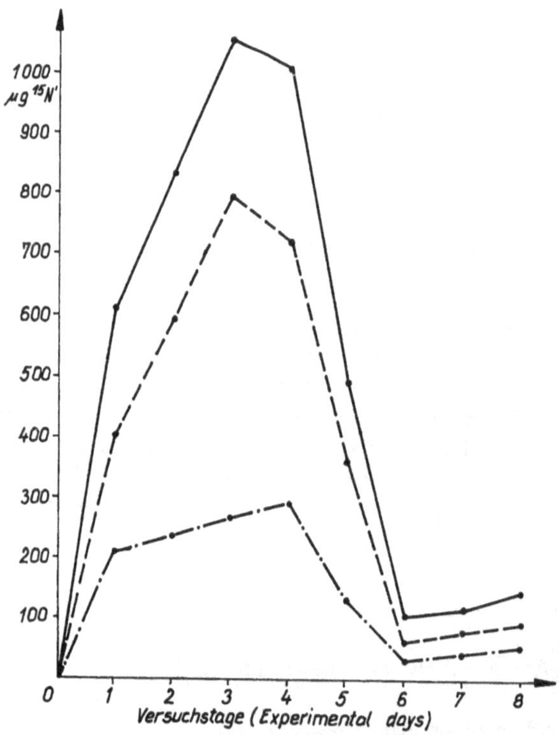

Abb. 4 (Fig. 4). Verlauf der $^{15}N'$-Exkretion mit Lysin (Course of $^{15}N'$ excretion with lysine). ——— gesamter Lysin-$^{15}N'$ (Total lysine-$^{15}N'$) – – – TCE-fällbarer Lysin-$^{15}N'$ (TCA-precipitable lysine-$^{15}N'$) —·— TCE-löslicher Lysin-$^{15}N'$ (TCA-soluble lysine-$^{15}N'$).

Vom 6. bis zum 8. Versuchstag wurden nur noch schwächer markierte Aminosäuren ausgeschieden, die vorwiegend aus sekretiertem Protein stammen dürften, da unverdauliche Futterbestandteile den Verdauungstrakt zu diesem Zeitpunkt passiert haben (Abb. 4, 5, 6).

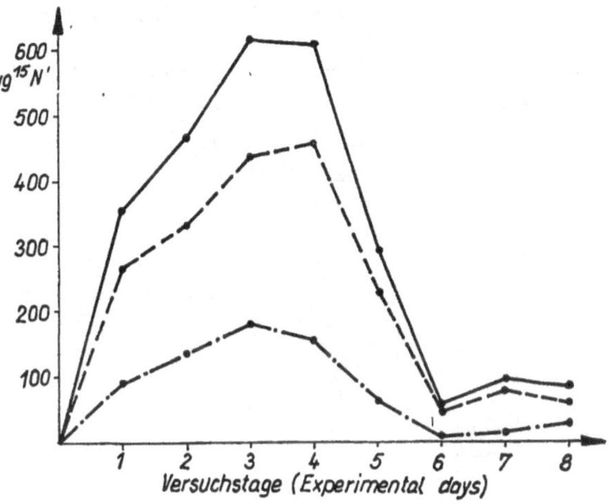

Abb. 5. (Fig. 5). Verlauf der $^{15}N'$-Exkretion mit Histidin (Course of $^{15}N'$ excretion with histidine). ——— Gesamter Histidin-$^{15}N'$ (Total histidine-$^{15}N'$) — — — TCE-fällbarer Histidin-$^{15}N'$ (TCA-precipitable histidine $^{15}N'$) —·— TCE-löslicher Histidin-$^{15}N'$ (TCA-soluble histidine-$^{15}N'$).

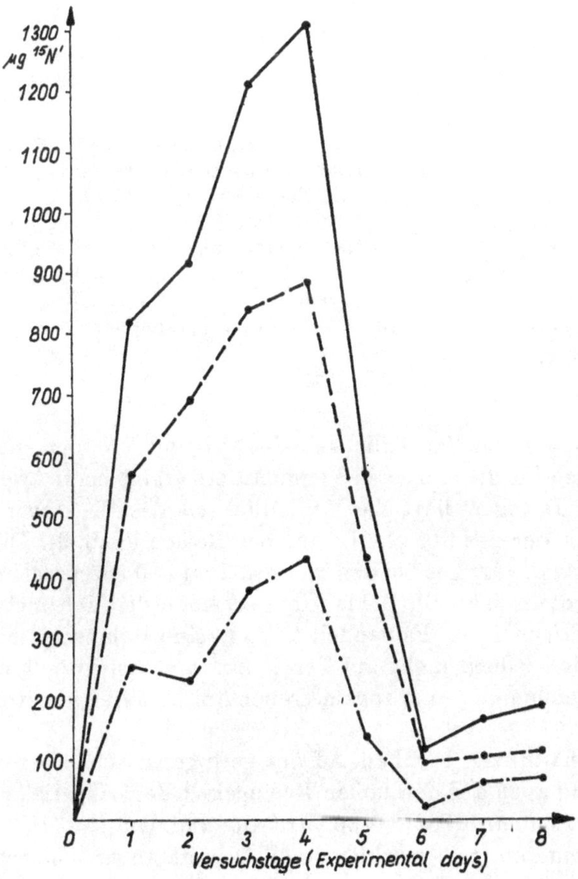

Abb. 6 (Fig. 6). Verlauf der $^{15}N'$-Exkretion mit Arginin (Course of $^{15}N'$ excretion with arginine). ——— gesamter Arginin-$^{15}N'$ (Total arginine-$^{15}N'$) — — — TCE-fällbarer Arginin-$^{15}N'$ (TCA-precipitable arginine-$^{15}N'$) —·— TCE-löslicher Arginin-$^{15}N'$ (TCA-soluble arginine-$^{15}N'$).

3.4.5. Scheinbare Verdaulichkeit des ^{14}N und $^{15}N'$ der basischen Aminosäuren

Vergleichend mit der Höhe der scheinbaren Verdaulichkeit des Rohproteins, konnten für Histidin und Arginin Werte, über jenen liegend, ermittelt werden, während sie für Lysin wesentlich darunter liegen. Die scheinbare Verdaulichkeit des $^{15}N'$-Lysins nimmt gegenüber den beiden anderen basischen Aminosäuren wesentlich schneller ab (Abb. 7).

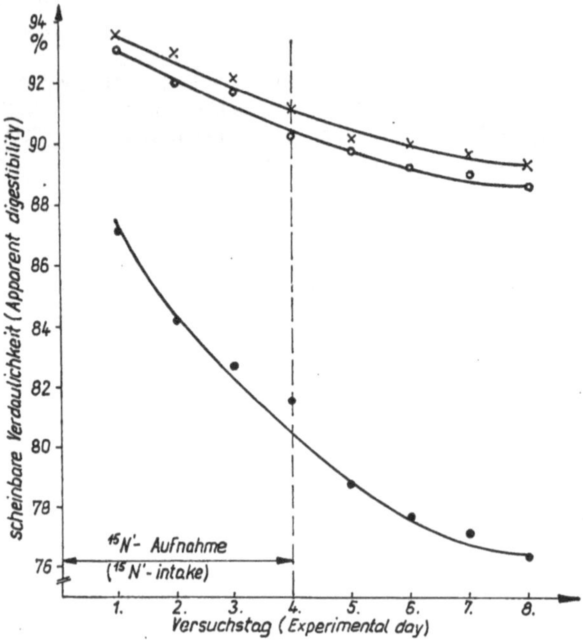

Abb. 7 (Fig. 7). Einfluß der Versuchsdauer auf die scheinbare Verdaulichkeit des $^{15}N'$ der basischen Aminosäuren (Influence of trial length on the apparent digestibility of the $^{15}N'$ of basic amino acids). ●●● Lysin (Lysine) ○○○ Histidin (Histidine) ××× Arginin (Arginine).

Ein Vergleich zwischen der scheinbaren Verdaulichkeit des ^{14}N und $^{15}N'$ der entsprechenden basischen Aminosäuren für die einzelnen Versuchstiere ergibt beim Arginin keine Unterschiede (Tab. 9). Dagegen liegt die Verdaulichkeit des $^{15}N'$-Lysins des Weizens im Mittel etwas unter der des übrigen Lysins der Ration (Tab. 9). Die auffällig niedrigen Verdauungswerte des Lysins bei den Hennen 2 und 10 entsprechen dem hohen Lysingehalt im Kotprotein (Tab. 6). Beide Tiere scheiden deutlich mehr ^{14}N und $^{15}N'$ im Kot aus als die übrigen Tiere. Es handelt sich um eine Malabsorption unbekannter Genese. Sie wirkt sich jedoch nicht auf den Aminosäurenstoffwechsel und die Legeleistung aus, da alle Hennen mit einer angemessenen Aminosäurengarnitur versorgt wurden.

Die Veränderungen in den Verhältnissen beruhen auf der geringeren scheinbaren Verdaulichkeit des Lysins. Sie sind auch auf den hohen Lysingehalt des bakteriellen Eiweißes zurückzuführen (PARSONS u. a., 1982). Von HENNIG und GRUHN (1978) wurden bei Verfütterung einer anderen, mit markiertem Stickstoff angereicherten Weizensorte Relativwerte für den Kot ermittelt, die mit den unsrigen weitgehend übereinstimmen, obwohl das Verhältnis des $^{15}N'$ zwischen Arginin und Lysin bzw. Arginin und Histidin im Futter breiter ist (Tab. 10).

Tabelle 9 (Table 9)
Scheinbare Verdaulichkeit des Stickstoffes mit natürlicher isotoper Häufigkeit und des schweren Stickstoffes von Lysin, Histidin und Arginin der einzelnen Hennen (in %)
(Apparent digestibility of nitrogen with natural isotopic frequency and of the heavy nitrogen of lysine, histidine and arginine in per cent)

Hennen-Nr. (Number of hen)	Versuchszeit, Tage (Experimental period, days)	Lysin (Lysine)		Histidin (Histidine)		Arginin (Arginine)	
		^{14}N	$^{15}N'$	^{14}N	$^{15}N'$	^{14}N	$^{15}N'$
1	4	82,5	82,4	86,1	91,2	89,1	90,8
2	4	72,6	72,1	80,8	86,2	86,6	89,2
3	4	82,4	83,2	87,0	91,8	90,2	91,4
4	5	80,3	77,7	84,6	89,8	89,0	89,1
5	5	81,4	79,3	85,5	88,7	88,2	89,7
6	5	82,7	83,5	88,8	92,3	91,1	93,2
7	6	82,6	79,4	86,8	89,4	88,8	91,0
8	6	82,9	78,8	87,8	89,4	90,0	89,3
9	6	84,2	82,3	88,4	91,7	91,0	90,6
10	8	73,1	74,3	82,6	83,5	87,9	84,4
11	8	78,4	75,5	84,7	85,5	88,7	88,5
12	8	81,0	77,5	88,0	89,4	91,1	91,4

Tabelle 10 (Table 10)
Vergleich der Verhältnisse der $^{15}N'$-Mengen der basischen Aminosäuren zwischen Kot und Futter
(Comparison of the relations of $^{15}N'$-amounts of basic amino acids in faeces and rations)

Aminosäuren (Amino acids)	Futter (Ration)	Kot (Faeces)	Futter (Ration) (HENNIG und GRUHN, 1978)	Kot (Faeces) (HENNIG und GRUHN, 1978)
Histidin : Lysin (Histidine : lysine)	1,19	0,59	1,13	0,58
Arginin : Lysin (Arginine : lysine)	2,65	1,22	3,28	1,23
Arginin : Histidin (Arginine : histidine)	2,23	2,05	2,89	2,12

Für die scheinbare Verdaulichkeit der basischen Aminosäuren des ^{15}N-markierten Weizens können folgende Werte errechnet werden:

Lysin 80,4 %, Histidin 90,8 % und Arginin 90,2 %.

Diese Werte repräsentieren ebenso wie beim Gesamt-$^{15}N'$ das Mittel der 12 Hennen am 3. und 4. Versuchstag, wo quasi-stationäre Verhältnisse angenommen werden können (Abb. 7). Für den $^{15}N'$ der basischen Aminosäuren wurden von HENNIG und GRUHN

(1978) mit einer anderen Weizensorte im wesentlichen die gleichen Werte ermittelt. Sie betrugen jeweils 80,3 %, 89,5 % und 92,2 %. Somit konnte mit Hilfe der Markierung für den Weizen eine hohe Verdaulichkeit des Proteins und der basischen Aminosäuren nachgewiesen werden.

Zusammenfassung

12 kolostomierte Legehennen erhielten 4 Tage mit einer produktionsüblichen Ration markierten Weizen mit 14,37 Atom-% ^{15}N Überschuß ($^{15}N'$). Die Markierung der basischen Aminosäuren betrug für Lysin 13,58 Atom-%, für Histidin 14,38 Atom-% und für Arginin 13,63 Atom-% $^{15}N'$. Jeweils 3 Tiere wurden 12 h, 36 h, 60 h bzw. 108 h nach der letzten ^{15}N-Gabe geschlachtet. Während der gesamten Versuchszeit erfolgte von den einzelnen Hennen täglich die Bestimmung des $^{15}N'$ im Gesamt-N und in der N-Fraktion nichteiweißartiger Herkunft sowie der basischen Aminosäuren des Kotes.

Das Rohprotein des Kotes enthielt im Mittel 5,45 % Lysin, 2,32 % Histidin und 3,68 % Arginin; das Reinprotein des Kotes enthielt entsprechend 5,43 % Lysin, 2,32 % Histidin und 4,07 % Arginin. Der Anteil des TCE-löslichen N am Gesamt-N des Kotes beträgt am dritten und vierten Versuchstag ein Drittel und für den $^{15}N'$ 28 %. Der mittlere Atom-% $^{15}N'$ der Proteinfraktion beträgt 3,48 Atom-% $^{15}N'$ und der der Nichteiweiß-N-Fraktion des Kotes 2,93 Atom-% $^{15}N'$. Die scheinbare Verdaulichkeit des ^{14}N der Ration liegt im Mittel bei 82,8 % und die des Weizen-$^{15}N'$ bei 87,5 %. Der mittlere Anteil der im Proteinverband des Kotes vorliegenden basischen Aminosäuren macht für Lysin-$^{15}N'$ 70,9 % aus. Die Verdaulichkeit der ^{15}N-markierten Aminosäuren beträgt für Lysin 80,4 %, Histidin 90,8 % und für Arginin 90,2 %.

Резюме

К. Грун и Г. Ярайс

Динамика обменов аминокислот и протеина кур-несушек после аппликации меченого ^{15}N пшеничного протеина. 2-ое сообщ.: Выделение ^{15}N вместе с азотом и основными аминокислотами кала

12 колостомированных кур-несушек получили в течение 4 дней вместе с нормальным хозяйственным рационом меченую пшеницу с 14,37 атом-% избытка ^{15}N ($^{15}N'$). Мечение основных аминокислот было у лизина 13,58 атом-% $^{15}N'$, у гистидина 14,38 атом-% $^{15'}N$ и у аргинина 13,63 атом-% $^{15}N'$. Затем убились по 3 курицам 12, 36, 60 или 108 часов после последного введения ^{15}N. Во время целого опыта анализировался ежедневно кал каждой курицы для определения тяжёлого азота в общем азоте, в азотной фракции небелкового происхождения и в основных аминокислотах.

Сырой протеин кала содержал в среднем 5,45 % лизина, 2,32 % гистидина и 3,68 % аргинина, а чистый протеин кала содержал соответственно 5,43 % лизина, 2,32 % гистидина и 4,07 % аргинина. Доля в ТХУК растворимого азота кала составила на третий и четвёртый подопытный день 1/3 и 28 % для $^{15}N'$. Средний избыток атом-% ^{15}N ($^{15}N'$) протеиновой фракции составил 3,48 атом-% $^{15}N'$ и относительно небелковой азотистой фракции кала 2,93 атом-% $^{15}N'$. Видимая переваримость ^{14}N рациона была в среднем 82,8 %, а для $^{15}N'$ пшеницы определились 87,5 %. Средняя доля основных аминокислот протеина кала составила для $^{15}N'$-лизина 70,9 %. Переваримость меченых ^{15}N аминокилот составила для лизина 80,4 %, для гистидина 90,8 % и для аргинина 90,2 %

Summary

K. Gruhn and G. Jahreis

Dynamics of the amino acid and protein metabolism of laying hens after the application of ^{15}N labelled wheat protein. 2. ^{15}N excretion with the nitrogen and the basic amino acids of faeces

Over 4 days 12 colostomized laying hens received together with a commercial ration labelled wheat with a ^{15}N excress ($^{15}N'$) of 14.37 atom-%. The labelling of the basic amino acids amounted to 13.58 atom-% for lysine, to 14.38 atom-% for histidine and to 13.63 atom-% $^{15}N'$ for arginine. 3 animals each were butchered 12 h, 36 h, 60 h and 108 h resp. after the last application of ^{15}N. The heavy nitrogen in the total N and in the N fraction of non-protein origin as well as in the basic amino acids in faeces was daily determined for the individual hens in the total experimental period.

On average the crude protein of faeces contained 5.45 % lysine, 2.32 % histidine and 3.68 % arginine: the protein of faeces correspondingly contained 5.43 % lysine, 2.32 % histidine and 4.07 % arginine. The quota of TCA soluble N in the total N of faeces amounts to one third on the 3rd und 4th days of the experiment and that of $^{15}N'$ to 28 %. The average atom-% $^{15}N'$ of the protein fraction is 3.48 atom-% $^{15}N'$ and that of the non-protein N fraction of faeces 2.93 atom-% $^{15}N'$. The apparent digestibility of the ^{14}N of the ration on average amounts to 82.8 % and that of the wheat $^{15}N'$ to 87.5 %. The average quota of the basic amino acids in the protein compounds of faeces amounts to 70.9 % for lysine $^{15}N'$, 73.7 % for histidine $^{15}N'$ and 70.3 % for arginine $^{15}N'$. The digestibility of the ^{15}N labelled amino acids amounts to 80.4 % for lysine, 90.8 % for histidine and 90.2 % for arginine.

Literaturverzeichnis

[1] Armstrong, F. B., S. Margen and H. Tarver: Proc. Soc. Exp. Biol. Med. **103**, 592 (1960)
[2] Bergner, U., H. Bergner und O. Simon: Arch. Tierernähr. **26**, 613 (1976)
[3] Bird, F. H.: Fed. Proc. **27**, 1194 (1968)
[4] Campbell, R. M., D. P. Cuthbertson, W. Mackie, A. S. McFarlane, A. T. Phillipson and S. Sudsaneh: J. Physiol. **158**, 113 (1961)
[5] Crompton, D. W. T. and M. C. Nesheim: J. Nutrit. **99**, 43 (1969)
[6] Figarella, C.: Arch. Franc. Malad. Appar. Dig. **62**, 337 (1973)
[7] Glass, G. B. J., and A. Ishimori: Amer. J. Dig. Dis. **6**, 103 (1961)
[8] Gruhn, K.: Arch. Tierernähr. **24**, 85 (1974)
[9] Gruhn, K., und G. Jahreis: Monatsh. Veterinärmed. **29**, 774 (1974)
[10] Hennig, A., G. Richter und K. Gruhn: Arch. Tierernähr. **25**, 195 (1975)

[11] HENNIG, A., und K. GRUHN: Arch. Tierernähr. **28**, 519 (1978)
[12] HENNIG, A., K. GRUHN und E. KIRCHNER: Arch. Tierernähr. **37**, 299 (1987)
[13] HOFFMANN M., G. GEBHARDT und R. KÖHLER: Arch. Tierernähr. **22**, 267 (1972)
[14] JAHREIS, G., und K. GRUHN: Arch. Tierernähr. **29**, 569 (1979)
[15] KIRCHNER, E., und K. GRUHN: Nahrung **29**, 703 (1985)
[16] MUNRO, H. N.: General aspects of the regulation of protein metabolism by diet and hormones. In: H. N. MUNRO and J. B. ALLISON: Mammalian protein metabolism. Academic Press, New York and London, Vol. I, 384 ff (1964)
[17] NASSET, E. S., and J. S. JU: J. Nutrit. **74**, 461 (1961)
[18] PARSONS, C. M., L. M. POTTER, R. D. BROWN, jr., T. D. WILKINS and B. A. BLISS: Poultry Sci. **61**, 925 (1982)
[19] PAYNE, W. L., G. F. COMBS, R. R. KIFER and D. G. SNYDER: Fed. Proc. **27**, 1199 (1968)
[20] WIESEMÜLLER, W.: Empfehlungen zur Durchführung von Fütterungsversuchen. Hochschulstudium, Agraringenieurwesen – Tierproduktion, Karl-Marx-Univ. Leipzig, Sektion Tierproduktion und Veterinärmedizin (1983)
[21] ZIMMER, M., H. BERGNER und O. SIMON: Arch. Tierernähr. **25**, 311 (1975)

Eingegangen: 21. August 1985

Anschriften der Autoren:

Dr. sc. agr. K. GRUHN und
Dr. agr. G. JAHREIS
Sektion Tierproduktion u. Veterinärmedizin
Karl-Marx-Universität Leipzig
Wissenschaftsbereich Tierernährungschemie
Dornburger Str. 24
Jena
DDR - 6900

Arch. Anim. Nutr., Berlin 37 (1987) 6, 521–531

Sektion Tierproduktion der Wilhelm-Pieck-Universität Rostock,
Wissenschaftsbereich Tierernährung
(Leiter: Prof. Dr. sc. agr. S. POPPE)[2]
Instituto de Ciencia Animal Habana
(Direktor: Dr. Arabel ELIAS)[1]

M. VALDIVIE[1] und S. POPPE[2]

Untersuchungen zur Energie- und Proteinkonzentration von Broilerrationen in Kuba

4. Mitteilung

Weibliche Broiler im Sommer

1. Einleitung

Die vorliegenden Untersuchungen mit weiblichen Broilern der Rasse White Plymouth Rock wurden durchgeführt, um die günstigsten Energie- und Proteinkonzentrationen der Rationen für diese Tiere unter den Bedingungen des kubanischen Sommers zu ermitteln. Außerdem sollte das Verhalten der weiblichen Broiler im Winter (VALDIVIE u. a., 1987b) und das Verhalten der männlichen Broiler im Sommer (VALDIVIE u. a., 1987c) mit den vorliegenden Ergebnissen verglichen werden, um mögliche jahreszeitliche Einflüsse zu quantifizieren. Außerdem sollten evtl. Geschlechtsdifferenzen dieser Broiler während der Aufzucht im Sommer erfaßt werden.

2. Material und Methoden

Mit insgesamt 1900 weiblichen Broilern der Rasse White Plymouth Rock wurden in den ersten 56. Lebenstagen in 16 Versuchsgruppen vier Energiekonzentrationen (10,5; 11,5; 12,6 und 13,6 MJ UE/kg und vier Rohproteinkonzentrationen (15,0; 17,5; 20,0 und 22,5 % RP) geprüft. Die Tiere wurden in Käfigen gehalten und waren ab 15. Lebenstag den natürlichen Sommertemperaturen in Kuba direkt ausgesetzt. Da jede Versuchsgruppe mit 6 Wiederholungen durchgeführt wurde, konnten die Ergebnisse varianzanalytisch verrechnet werden.

Im übrigen wurde in diesem Versuch methodisch genauso verfahren, wie das von VALDIVIE u. a. (1986) beschrieben wurde.

3. Versuchsergebnisse

3.1. Gesundheitszustand der Versuchstiere

Die Versuchstiere zeigten während des Versuches keinerlei Krankheitssymptome. Tierverluste traten kaum auf, sie schwankten zwischen 0 und 2 Tieren je Gruppe. Es traten keine Verlusthäufungen bei bestimmten Rohprotein- bzw. Energieniveaus auf. Die Tiere der Versuchsgruppe mit 13,6 MJ UE und 15,0 % RP zeigten eine ungenügende Befiederung als Folge der Imbalanz zwischen Energie und Rohprotein bzw. den Aminosäuren dieser Ration.

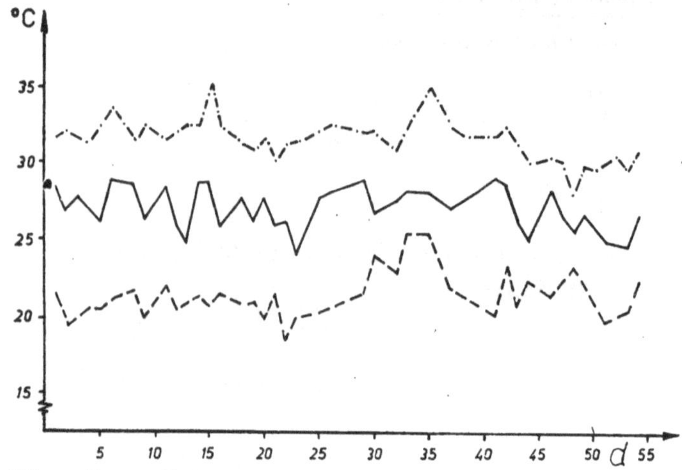

Abb. 1 (Fig. 1). Lufttemperatur (Air temperature)
—·— maximale Temperatur (Maximal temperature)
——— mittlere Temperatur (Medium temperature)
– – – minimale Temperatur (Minimal temperature)

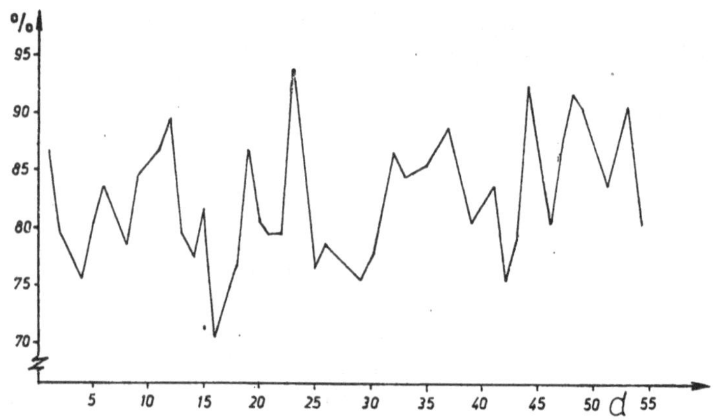

Abb. 2 (Fig. 2). Relative Luftfeuchtigkeit (Relative humidity)

Tabelle 1 (Table 1)
Futterverzehr vom 1.–56. Lebenstag (g/Tier)
(Feed intake from the 1st to 56th day of life, g/animal)

RP (%) (CP, %) UE (ME)/kg	15,0	17,5	20,0	22,5
10,5 MJ	2679 a	2719 ab	2995 bcd	3170 d
11,6 MJ	2988 bcd	3131 d	2944 abcd	3108 cd
12,6 MJ	2988 bcd	2910 bcd	2937 abcd	2974 bcd
13,6 MJ	2723 ab	3098 cd	2852 abc	2722 ab

$SE \pm 83$ $P < 0{,}001$

3.2. Futterverzehr

Es konnte kein linearer Einfluß der Energie- bzw. Rohproteinkonzentration der Ration auf den Futterverzehr der weiblichen Broiler im Sommer festgestellt werden. Die Mittelwerte des Futterverzehrs vom 1.–56. Lebenstag sind in Tab. 1 dargestellt.

Der Futterverzehr der Broiler war sehr niedrig.

3.3. Energieaufnahme

Die entsprechenden Werte für die Energieaufnahme sind in Tabelle 2 dargestellt.

Tabelle 2 (Table 2)
Energieaufnahme vom 1.–56. Lebenstag (MJ)
(Energy intake from the 1st to 56th day of life, MJ)

RP (%) (CP, %) UE (ME)/kg	15,0	17,5	20,0	22,5
10,5 MJ	28,64 g	28,08 g	31,50 f	32,66 ef
11,5 MJ	33,24 e	35,71 d	33,51 e	35,92 cd
12,6 MJ	37,39 abc	37,41 abc	37,78 ab	37,62 ab
13,6 MJ	37,75 ab	38,17 a	38,85 a	36,61 bcd
	SE ±0,52	*P* <0,05		

Aus Tab. 2 ist ersichtlich, daß bei isonitrogenen Rationen mit steigender Energiekonzentration der Energieverzehr in der Tendenz erhöht wird.

3.4. Rohproteinaufnahme

Die Rohproteinaufnahme für den Gesamtversuch ist in Tab. 3 dargestellt.

Aus Tab. 3 ist zu ersehen, daß bei isoenergetischen Rationen mit steigender Rohproteinkonzentration der Rohproteinverzehr ansteigt.

Tabelle 3 (Table 3)
Rohproteinaufnahme vom 1.–56. Lebenstag (g/Tier)
(Crude protein intake from the 1st to 56th day of life, g/animal)

RP (%) (CP, %) UE (ME)/kg	15,0	17,5	20,0	22,5
10,5 MJ	400 a	476 bc	596 gh	713 j
11,5 MJ	448 b	547 ef	576 fgh	699 ij
12,6 MJ	448 b	523 de	587 gh	669 i
13,6 MJ	408 e	501 cd	570 fg	612 h
	SE ±11	*P* <0,001		

3.5. Lebendmasse und Lebendmassezunahme

In Tab. 4 sind die mittleren Lebendmassen der Versuchstiere am 28. Lebenstag dargestellt.

Tabelle 4 (Table 4)
Lebendmasse am 28. Lebenstag (g/Tier)
(Live weight at the 28th day of life, g/animal)

RP (%) (CP, %) UE (ME)/kg	15,0	17,5	20,0	22,5
10,5 MJ	277 a	361 b	421 de	481 gh
11,5 MJ	358 b	442 ef	384 bc	486 h
12,6 MJ	399 cd	449 f	491 h	533 i
13,6 MJ	400 cd	457 fg	498 h	499 h
	$SE \pm 9$	$P < 0{,}001$		

Durch die Erhöhung der Rohproteinkonzentration wird bei der niedrigsten Energiekonzentration die Lebendmasse am 28. Lebenstag erhöht, dies trifft auch für die Gruppen mit 12,6 MJ UE zu. Beim Energieniveau von 11,5 MJ UE wird die höchste Lebendmasse mit 22,5 % RP erreicht, während beim Energieniveau von 13,6 MJ UE bei 20 bzw. 22,5 % RP die höchsten Lebendmassen gefunden wurden.

Diese Ergebnisse zeigen, daß die weiblichen Broiler im Sommer bis zum 28. Lebenstag höhere Rohproteinkonzentrationen im Futter benötigen, als die weiblichen Tiere im Winter, obwohl das Wachstum der Tiere im Sommer niedriger als im Winter war. Bei den Tieren der Rohproteinniveaus von 15 bis 20 % wurden die höchsten Lebendmassen bei 12,6 buw. 13,6 MJ UE gefunden, bei der Rohproteinstufe von 17,5 % wiesen die Tiere der Gruppen mit 11,5; 12,6 bzw. 13,6 MJ UE die höchsten Lebendmassen auf. Beim Rohproteinniveau von 22,5 % wurde die höchste Lebendmasse bei 12,6 MJ UE gefunden. Die Resultate zeigen, daß mit einer Energiekonzentration von 12,6 MJ UE innerhalb einer Rohproteinstufe (15–22,5 %) die höchst möglichen Lebendmassen am 28. Lebenstag erreicht werden können. Die höchsten Lebendmassen am 28. Lebenstag hatten die Tiere der Gruppe mit 12,6 MJ UE und 22,5 % RP. Die im 2. Mastabschnitt erreichten Lebendmassezunahmen sind Tab. 5 zu entnehmen.

Tabelle 5 (Table 5)
Lebendmassezunahme vom 29.–56. Lebenstag (g/Tier)
(Weight gain from the 29th to 56th day of life, g/animal)

RP (%) (CP, %) UE (ME)/kg	15,0	17,5	20,0	22,5
10,5 MJ	596 c	718 ab	763 a	760 a
11,5 MJ	694 b	768 a	724 ab	752 ab
12,6 MJ	714 ab	724 ab	714 ab	755 ab
13,6 MJ	743 ab	778 a	765 a	740 ab
	$SE \pm 12$	$P < 0{,}05$		

Diese Lebendmassezunahmen sind sehr niedrig, sie liegen zwischen 596 und 778 g je Tier. In 14 von 16 Versuchsgruppen wurden maximale Lebendmassezunahmen von 714 bis 778 g erreicht, die sich nicht signifikant unterschieden.

In Tab. 6 sind die Lebendmassen der Tiere am 56. Lebenstag dargestellt.

Tabelle 6 (Table 6)
Lebendmasse am 56. Lebenstag (g/Tier)
(Live weight at the 56th day of life, g/animal)

RP (%) (CP, %) UE (ME)/kg	15,0	17,5	20,0	22,5
10,5 MJ	906 a	1106 bc	1216 efg	1272 fgh
11,5 MJ	1083 b	1243 efg	1141 bcd	1270 fgh
12,6 MJ	1143 bcd	1204 def	1236 efg	1321 h
13,6 MJ	1176 cde	1266 fgh	1293 gh	1269 fgh
	$SE \pm 24$	$P < 0{,}001$		

Die höchsten Lebendmassen am Versuchsende wurden von den Gruppen mit 22,5 % RP und den Gruppen mit 13,6 MJ UE und 20 bzw. 17,5 % RP erreicht.

Wenn mit einem 2- oder 3-phasischen Fütterungssystem gearbeitet worden wäre, hätte mit größerer Sicherheit die für die weiblichen Broiler im Sommer notwendige Energie- bzw. Rohproteinkonzentration abgeleitet werden können. Die vorliegenden Ergebnisse zeigen die Möglichkeit der Reduzierung der Rohproteinkonzentration im Futter im 2. Mastabschnitt.

3.6. Futteraufwand

In Tab. 7 sind die mittleren Futteraufwandszahlen für die einzelnen Gruppen dargestellt.

Der niedrigste Futteraufwand wurde in den einzelnen Rohproteinniveaus immer bei der höchsten Energiekonzentration erreicht. Beim Rohproteinniveau von 22,5 % wurde auch schon mit 12,6 MJ UE ein akzeptabler Futteraufwand erzielt.

Der niedrigste Futteraufwand wurde mit 13,6 MJ UE und 22 % RP erreicht. In den einzelnen Energiestufen lag beim Rohproteinniveau von 15,0 % immer der höchste Energieaufwand vor.

Tabelle 7 (Table 7)
Futteraufwand vom 1.–56. Lebenstag
(Feed efficiency from the 1st to 56th day of life)

RP (%) (CP, %) UE (ME)/kg	15,0	17,5	20,0	22,5
10,5 MJ	3,17 a	2,49 e	2,55 cde	2,52 de
11,5 MJ	2,75 b	2,57 cde	2,63 bcd	2,52 de
12,6 MJ	2,68 b	2,54 cde	2,49 e	2,33 fg
13,6 MJ	2,43 ef	2,29 g	2,26 g	2,17 g
	$SE \pm 0{,}07$	$P < 0{,}05$		

3.7. Schlachtmassenausbeute und Abdominalfett

In Tab. 8 ist die Schlachtmassenausbeute am Versuchsende dargestellt.

Tabelle 8 (Table 8)
Schlachtmassenausbeute am 56. Lebenstag (%)
(Carcass yield at the 56th day of life, %)

RP (%) (CP, %) UE (ME)/kg	15,0	17,5	20,0	22,5
10,5 MJ	65,3 a	68,3 bcde	70,9 b	67,8 bcd
11,5 MJ	70,6 ef	68,0 bcd	66,3 ab	69,1 cdef
12,6 MJ	68,6 cdef	67,8 bcd	70,0 def	70,0 def
13,6 MJ	68,4 bcde	67,5 bc	70,5 ef	70,0 def
	$SE \pm 0{,}07$	$P < 0{,}001$		

Die Schlachtmassenausbeute schwankte zwischen 65,3 und 70,9 %. Schlachtmassenausbeuten mit Mittelwerten zwischen 70 % und 70,9 % wurden mit den Rationen von 13,6 MJ UE und 20 bzw. 22,5 % RP, 12,6 MJ UE und 20 bzw. 22,5 % RP, 11,5 MJ UE und 15 % RP und 10,5 MJ UE und 20 % RP erreicht. Die niedrigste Schlachtmassenausbeute wurde bei der Ration 10,4 MJ UE und 15 % RP gefunden, die gleichzeitig zur niedrigsten Lebendmasse führte. Alle übrigen Gruppen wiesen Schlachtmassenausbeuten zwischen 67,8 und 69,1 % auf.

Die niedrigste Schlachtmassenausbeute der weiblichen Broiler im Sommer (65,3 %) als auch die Werte unter 68,4 % liegen tiefer als diese Werte in den vorangegangenen 3 Experimenten. In 14 Fällen der 16 Vergleichsvarianten wiesen die weiblichen Broiler im Sommer die niedrigsten Schlachtmassenausbeuten in allen 4 Experimenten auf. Die Ursache dafür liegt in der niedrigen Lebendmasse am 56. Lebenstag in diesem Versuch. In Tab. 9 sind die Mittelwerte der Abdominalfettmengen dargestellt.

Tabelle 9 (Table 9)
Abdominalfett am 56. Lebenstag (g/Tier)
(Abdominal fat at the 56th day of life, g/animal)

RP (%) (CP, %) UE (ME)/kg	15,0	17,5	20,0	22,5
10,5 MJ	14,0 d	19,1 cd	20,3 c	16,2 cd
11,5 MJ	35,3 a	31,4 ab	19,4 cd	26,2 b
12,6 MJ	29,3 ab	32,9 ab	29,2 ab	18,2 cd
13,6 MJ	36,3 a	38,6 a	25,0 b	23,4 b
	$SE \pm 3{,}0$	$P < 0{,}01$		

Die Abdominalfettmengen variieren zwischen 14 und 38,6 g je Tier. Die Gruppen mit 11,5, 12,6 und 13,6 MJ UE wiesen bei 15 bzw. 17,5 % RP die höchsten Abdominalfettmengen auf. Hohe Abdominalfettmengen werden auch bei den Tieren der Gruppe mit 12,6 MJ UE und 20 % RP gefunden. Diese Befunde stimmen mit der

Literatur überein, daß eine Erhöhung der Energiekonzentration in Verbindung mit einer Verminderung der Proteinkonzentration in der Ration zu höheren Abdominalfettmengen führt. Die niedrigsten Abdominalfettmengen sind in den 4 Gruppen der untersten Energiestufe (10,5 MJ UE) und bei den Rationen mit 11,5 MJ UE und 20 % RP sowie 12,6 MJ UE mit 22,5 % RP zu finden. Damit wird deutlich, daß die Energiekonzentration der Ration einen großen Einfluß auf den Ansatz des Abdominalfettes hat.

3.8. Körperprotein

Die Körperproteinmengen am Versuchsende sind in Tab. 10 dargestellt.

Tabelle 10 (Table 10)
Körperproteinmengen am 56. Lebenstag (g/Tier)
(Amount of body protein at the 56th day of life, g/animal)

RP (%) (CP, %) UE (ME)/kg	15,0	17,5	20,0	22,5
10,5 MJ	157 f	183 e	215 bc	229 ab
11,5 MJ	287 de	222 b	202 c	231 ab
12,6 MJ	199 cd	206 c	223 b	242 a
13,6 MJ	206 c	226 b	242 a	229 ab
	SE ±0,2	*P* <0,05		

Aus Tab. 10 ist ersichtlich, daß in den einzelnen Energiestufen mit steigender Rohproteinkonzentration sich die Körperproteinmengen erhöhen, mit Ausnahme der Gruppen mit 13,6 MJ UE und 22,5 % RP und 11,5 MJ UE mit 20 % RP. Die höchsten Körperproteinmengen wurden bei den 4 Gruppen mit 22,5 % RP und der Gruppe mit 13,6 MJ UE und 20 % RP gefunden.

3.9. Proteinverwertung

Die Mittelwerte der Proteinverwertung für den gesamten Mastabschnitt sind in Tabelle 13 dargestellt.

Bei der Betrachtung der Mittelwerte wird die Tendenz deutlich, daß mit steigender Rohproteinkonzentration in der Ration und damit Erhöhung des Rohproteinverzehrs

Tabelle 11 (Table 11)
Proteinverwertung vom 1.–56. Lebenstag (%)
(Protein efficiency from the 1st to 56th day of life, %)

RP (%) (CP, %) UE (ME)/kg	15,0	17,5	20,0	22,5
10,5 MJ	37,9 f	37,8 f	35,3 fg	31,8 h
11,5 MJ	41,2 cd	39,9 d	34,1 gh	32,4 h
12,6 MJ	43,5 bc	38,2 e	37,1 f	35,4 fg
13,6 MJ	48,1 a	44,2 b	41,8 bcd	36,9 f
	SE ±0,84	*P* <0,05		

sich die Proteinverwertung vermindert, weil der Körperproteinansatz sich nicht proportional erhöht. In den einzelnen Rohproteinstufen finden sich bei der Energiekonzentration von 13,6 MJ UE die höchste und bei der Energiekonzentration von 10,5 MJ UE die niedrigste Proteinverwertung. Die Proteinverwertung der Gruppen mit 11,5 und 12,6 MJ UE ist innerhalb der einzelnen Rohproteinniveaus in einigen Fällen signifikant unterschiedlich und in anderen Fällen nicht verschieden voneinander.

3.10. Körperfett

In Tab. 12 sind die Körperfettmengen der Versuchstiere am Versuchsende dargestellt.

Tabelle 12 (Table 12)
Körperfettmenge am 56. Lebenstag (g)
(Amount of body fat at the 56th day of life, g)

RP (%) (CP, %) UE (ME)/kg	15,0	17,5	20,0	22,5
10,5 MJ	142 gh	168 de	153 fg	128 i
11,5 MJ	171 cd	166 def	164 cd	158 ef
12,6 MJ	175 cd	183 bc	176 cd	137 hi
13,6 MJ	195 ab	191 ab	197 a	191 ab

$SE \pm 0{,}2$ $P < 0{,}05$

Aus Tab. 12 ist zu ersehen, daß in den einzelnen Rohproteinniveaus mit steigender Energiekonzentration der Ration gleichzeitig der Körperfettgehalt ansteigt, mit Ausnahme der Gruppe mit 11,5 MJ UE und 17,5 % RP und der Gruppe mit 12,6 MJ UE und 22,5 % RP.

3.11. Energieverwertung

Bei der Energieverwertung traten keine linearen unabhängigen Effekte der unterschiedlichen Energie- und Rohproteinkonzentrationen auf. Es sind jedoch Interaktionen von Energie- und Rohproteinkonzentrationen des Futters auf die Energieverwertung vorhanden. In Tab. 13 ist die Energieverwertung für den gesamten Mastabschnitt dargestellt.

Tabelle 13 (Table 13)
Energieverwertung vom 1.–56. Lebenstag (%)
(Energy efficiency from the 1st to 56th day of life, %)

RP (%) (CP, %) UE (ME)/kg	15,0	17,5	20,0	22,5
10,5 MJ	30,2 gh	37,5 a	33,0 bc	30,9 defg
11,5 MJ	31,4 cdefg	30,9 defg	32,4 cd	30,5 efgh
12,6 MJ	29,0 hi	30,3 fgh	30,0 gh	27,7 i
13,6 MJ	32,0 cdef	32,3 cde	32,3 bcd	34,1 b

$SE \pm 0{,}6$ $P < 0{,}05$

Diskussion

Bei einem Vergleich des Verhaltens der männlichen und weiblichen Broiler im Sommer in Kuba (VALDIVIE und POPPE 1987 b) wird deutlich, daß die männlichen Tiere einen höheren Futterverzehr, eine höhere Aufnahme an Energie und Rohprotein als die weiblichen Tiere realisierten und dadurch eine höhere Lebendmasse und einen höheren Körperproteingehalt erreichten. Diese Befunde stimmen mit den Beobachtungen zwischen beiden Geschlechtern im Winter überein (VALDIVIE u. a., 1986; VALDIVIE und POPPE, 1987 a). Ähnliche Feststellungen treffen auch AJENJO (1964), RICHARD u. a. (1969), SUMMER u. a. (1972), FISHER (1980) und JACKSON u. a. (1982). Es sei betont, daß von den 14 vergleichbaren Gruppen, die weiblichen Tiere in 13 Fällen einen geringeren Futteraufwand und eine höhere Energieverwertung als die männlichen Tiere aufwiesen. Diese bessere Verwertung der Nährstoffe durch die weiblichen Tiere ist bedingt durch den extrem niedrigen Futterverzehr und ihre geringere Lebendmasse. Der jahreszeitliche Einfluß auf das Verhalten der weiblichen Broiler der Rasse White Plymouth Rock kann eingeschätzt werden, wenn die vorliegenden Ergebnisse mit denen aus der 2. Mitteilung dieser Serie verglichen werden (VALDIVIE und POPPE, 1987 a). Im Winter nahmen die weiblichen Broiler zwischen 15,7 und 36,4 % mehr Futter auf als im Sommer, dadurch realisierten sie im Winter eine um 11,1 bis 43,0 % höhere Lebendmasse. Außerdem war in allen Versuchsgruppen im Winter eine höhere Körperprotein- und Körperfettmasse bei den weiblichen Broilern als im Sommer gefunden worden. Dies stimmt auch überein mit den Feststellungen in der 3. Mitteilung (VALDIVIE und POPPE, 1987 b) bei einem Vergleich der männlichen und weiblichen Broiler im Winter. Ähnliche Befunde teilen auch SRURKIE (1965), SCOTT u. a. (1969), OLSON u. a. (1972), NRC (1977) und GONZALES u. a. (1980) mit.

Die weiblichen Broiler weisen im Sommer einen geringeren Futteraufwand auf als im Winter. Die Proteinverwertung war in 12 von 16 vergleichbaren Gruppen im Sommer höher als im Winter. Die Energieverwertung war im Sommer in allen 16 Gruppen höher als im Winter. Diese Befunde sind durch den außerordentlich niedrigen Futterverzehr und die niedrige Lebendmasse der Tiere bei diesen hohen Haltungstemperaturen zu erklären.

Zusammenfassung

Mit insgesamt 1900 weiblichen Broilern der Rasse White Plymouth Rock wurden in den ersten 56 Lebenstagen in 16 Versuchsgruppen vier Energiekonzentrationen (10,5; 11,5; 12,6 und 13,6 MJ UE/kg Futter) und vier Proteinkonzentrationen (15,0; 17,5; 20,0 und 22,5 % RP) geprüft. Die Tiere wurden in Käfigen gehalten und waren ab 15. Lebenstag den natürlichen Sommertemperaturen in Kuba direkt ausgesetzt. Da jede Versuchsgruppe mit 6 Wiederholungen durchgeführt wurde, konnten die Ergebnisse varianzanalytisch verrechnet werden. Bei einem Vergleich der männlichen und weiblichen Broiler im Sommer kann festgestellt werden, daß die weiblichen Tiere einen geringeren Verzehr an Futter, Energie und Rohprotein realisierten und geringere Lebendmassen erreichten als die männlichen Tiere. Die weiblichen Broiler nahmen im Winter zwischen 15,7 und 36,4 % mehr Futter und zwischen 11,1 und 43 % mehr an Lebendmasse zu als im Sommer. Es konnte gezeigt werden, daß maximale Lebendmassen der weiblichen Broiler im Sommer, wenn bei einem einphasischen Fütterungssystem Rationen mit 12,6 MJ UE und 22,5 % RP oder mit 13,6 MJ UE und 20 % RP gefüttert werden, erreichbar sind.

Резюме

М. Вальдивие и С. Поппе

Исследование по концентрации энергии и протеина в рационах птиц-бройлеров в Кубе. 4-ье сообщ.: ♀ бройлеры летом

Проводились опыты на всего 1900 ♀ птицах-бройлерах породы «*White Plymouth Rock*». Птицы разделились в первые 56 дней жизни в 16 опытные группы для изучения 4 различных концентраций энергии (10,5; 11,5; 12,6 и 13,6 МДж обменной энергии [ОЭ] на кг корма) и 4 различных концентраций сырого протеина (15,0; 17,5; 20,0 и 22,5 % СП). Птицы содержались в клетках, а с 15-ого для жизни прямо под условиями настоящего лета в Кубе. Каждая опытная группа повторялась 6 раз и, таким образом, возможно было вычисление данных с помощью вариационного анализа.

При сравнеии ♂ и ♀ бройлеров летом обнаружили, что ♀ птицы потребились по сравнению с ♂ птицами меньше корма, энергии и сырого протеина, а привесы были у ♀ птиц тоже ниже. ♀ бройлеры потребили зимой от 15,7 до 36,4 % больше корма и росли от 11,1 до 43 % лучше, чем летом. Показано, что получаются максимальные живые массы у ♀ бройлеров летом, если при однофазном режиме кормления птицам дадут рационы с 12,6 МДж ОЭ и 22,5 % СП или с 13,6 МДж ОЭ и 20 % СП.

Summary

M. Valdivie and S. Poppe

Studies on the energy and protein concentration in broiler rations in Cuba. 4. Female broilers in summer

A total of 1,900 female broilers of the variety White Plymouth Rock was tested with 4 energy concentrations (10.5, 11.5, 12.6 and 13.6 MJ metabolizable energy/kg feed) and 4 protein concentrations (15.0, 17.5, 20.0 and 22.5 % CP) in their first 56 days of life in 16 test groups. The animals were kept in cages and were directly exposed to the natural Cuban summer temperatures from their 15th day of life onwards. As every test group was run with 6 repetitions, the results could be variance analytically calculated. In a comparison of male and female broilers in summer one can state that the female animals achieved a lower intake of feed, energy and crude protein as well as a lower live weight than the male animals. In winter the female broilers consumed between 15.7 and 36.4 % more feed and achieved a live weight gain between 11.1 and 43 % higher than in summer. It could be shown that the maximum live weight of the female broilers could be achieved in summer if rations containing 12.6 MJ metabolizable energy and 20 % CP are fed in a one-phase feeeding system.

Literaturverzeichnis

[1] AJENJO, C.: Enciclopedia de Avicultura Madrid (1964)
[2] FISHER, C.: Protein Deposition in animals, Ed. by Butterworths (1980)
[3] GONZALEZ, A. und M. VALDIVIE: Forschungsbericht – ICA, Kuba (1980)
[4] JACKSON, S., J. D. SUMMERS und S. DEESOU: J. Poultry sci **61**, 2224 (1982)
[5] NRC: Nutrient requirements od domestic animal Nr. 1, Nutrient requirements of poultry (1977)
[6] OLSON, D. W., M. L. SUNDE und H. R. BIRG: J. Poultry Sci. 51, 1915 (1972)
[7] RICHARD, F. H. und M. ROUVIER: Ann. Gent. sel. Anim. **1**, 151 (1969)
[8] SCOTT, M. L., K. C. NESHEIM und R. I. YOUNG: Nutrition of the chicken. Ed. by Humphrey press, Geneva, New York (1969)
[9] SRURKIE, P. D.: Avian Physiology. Second edition. Ed. Cornell University, USA (1965)
[10] SUMMERS, J. D. und S. LEESON: Poultry Nutrition Handbook, Guelph, Ontario (1976)
[11] VALDIVIE, M., S. POPPE, HANNA MEIER und M. GABEL: Arch. Tierernähr. **35**, (1986)
[12] VALDIVIE, M. und S. POPPE: Arch. Tierernähr. **36**, 215 (1987 a)
[13] VALDIVIE, M. und S. POPPE: Arch. Tierernähr. **36**, 417 (1987 b)

Eingegangen: 5. Februar 1985

Anschrift der Autoren:

Prof. Dr. sc. S. POPPE
Wilhelm-Pieck-Universität Rostock
Sektion Tierproduktion
Wissenschaftsbereich Tierernährung
Justus-von-Liebig-Straße
Postfach 27–07
Rostock
2500
DDR

M. VALDIVIE
Republica de Cuba
Instituto de Ciencia Animal
Calle
Nuevo Vedado
La Habana

Arch. Anim. Nutr., Berlin 37 (1987) 6, 533–538

Institute of Commodity Science,
Academy of Economics
Cracow, Poland

MARIA KREŁOWSKA-KUŁAS

The effect of krill meal at lowered chitin contents in feed mixtures for fattening pigs on depot fat quality

1. Introduction

Research carried out so far that some authors show, that krill meal may replace expensive and deficit protein feeds used in the fattening of pigs (GLAPŚ et al., 1980; LEAT et al., 1964 and PASTUSZEWSKA, 1979). Chitin contents in the krill meal amounting to 4–5 % is to some degree a negative characteristic. Literature lacks information on the subject of using krill meal devoid of chitin contents in pigs feeding.

The effect of lipids in the diet on the physico-chemical properties of depot fat is well known (LEAT et al., 1964; PEZACKI et al. 1967). The composition of fatty acids and the degree of their unsaturation determine the technological and nutritional properties of fatty tissues (KOTARBIŃSKA and GROSZYK, 1977; PEZACKI et al., 1967).

The aim of the research was to determine the influence of fattening pigs feeding with mixture with krill meal at lowering chitin of about 50 % on the physicochemical properties of depot fat of fattening pigs.

2. Material and methods

The experiment was conducted on 60 pigs of White Large (Polish) breed with an initial body weight approx. 45 kg. The animals were divided into two experimental groups (15 ♀ and 15 ♂ in each group).

The experimental fattening was conducted until the animals achieved a body weight of approx. 120 kg.

The control group (K) was given mixture with "Provit" concentrate. In the experimental group (D) protein of "Provit" concentrate was replaced by protein of krill meal of the decreased 2.25 % chitin content (Table 1).

Samples of back fat and suet were collected from the right side of half carcass. The content of dry matter in back fat and suet were determined by the drying method (RUTKOWSKI and KRYGIER), and fat content by the extraction method of Soxhlet (RUTKOWSKI and KRYGIER).

In the fat obtained by the melting method at 95 °C, in tissues under analysis determinations refraction coefficient and melting point were determined by RUTKOWSKI and KRYGIER. The iodine number of fat was estimated by HANUS method (RUTKOWSKI and KRYGIER). The percent content of various fatty acids was determined by

Table 1

Composition of complete mixtures

Components %	Group K (Control group) Mixture Starter	Finisher	D (Experimental group) Starter	Finisher
"Prowit"-concentrate	16.0	12.0	–	–
Krill meal	–	–	14,0	10.0
Barley	56.5	60.5	58.5	62.5
Potato flakes	25.0	25.0	25.0	25.0
Fodder chalk	0.5	0.5	0.5	0.5
Fodder phosphate	1.0	1.0	1.0	1.0
Polfamiks	0.5	0.5	0.5	0.5
Fodder salt	0.5	0.5	0.5	0.5

the method of gas chromatography. Fat was extracted by BLIGHA und DYER (1959) method. The methyl esters of fatty acids were prepared according to Endress (1966).

The distribution of methyl esters was estimated on a gas chromatograph Pye Unicam 104, equipped with a flame–ionisation detector. For fatty acids separation were used: a glass column 210 cm filled 10 % EGSS on Chromosorb W 80–100 mesh, column temperature–200 °C, carrier gas-argon with a flow rate 30 ml/min.

The statistical calculations of significance of differences were made according to the principles given by RUSZCZYC (1978).

3. Results

Results of water and fat contents in the back fat and suet (Table 2) have shown that the back fat and suet of pigs of growing on D fed with the krill meal at low chitin level in complete mixtures contained a statistically significant high percentage of water and

Table 2

Coeficient of refraction, melting point, iodine number, content of fat and water in back fat and suet

	Water %	Fat %	Coefficient of refraction	Melting point °C	Iodine number
Back fat					
K	4.7 a	94.0 a	1.4587 a	36.82 A	59.35 A
D	5.6 b	91.8 b	1.4602 b	34.01 B	61.70 B
Suet					
K	3.6 a	94.0 a	1.4577 a	43.10 A	50.87 a
D	4.8 b	93.3 b	1.4586 b	39.92 B	52.11 b

a, b – values with different superscripts are significantly different $P < 0.05$
A, B – values with different superscripts are higly significantly different $P < 0.01$

Tabelle 3
Percent fatty acids content in back fat and suet

Fatty acids		Back fat Group K	Back fat Group D	Suet Group K	Suet Group D
$C_{10:0}$	$\bar{x}$	0.04	0.05	0.04	0.03
	s	0.01	0.02	0.02	0.01
$C_{12:0}$	$\bar{x}$	0.06	0.07	0.03	0.04
	s	0.01	0.02	0.01	0.02
$C_{14:0}$	$\bar{x}$	0.97	0.80	0.98	1,20
	s	0.40	0.35	0.25	0.30
$C_{15:0}$	$\bar{x}$	0.08	0.06	0.08	0.09
	s	0.02	0.01	0.03	0.02
$C_{16:0}$	$\bar{x}$	24.12 *A*	21.00 *B*	25.04	22.81
	s	1.53	1.40	1.09	1.18
$C_{16:1}$	$\bar{x}$	2.24	2.54	2.04	2.12
	s	0.56	0.60	0.40	0.48
$C_{17:0}$	$\bar{x}$	0.29 *A*	0.82 *B*	0.12 *A*	0.80 *B*
	s	0.05	0.07	0.03	0.05
$C_{17:1}$	$\bar{x}$	0.12 *A*	0.59 *B*	0.06 *A*	0.28 *B*
	s	0.02	0.04	0.02	0.04
$C_{18:0}$	$\bar{x}$	12.40 *a*	14.79 *b*	22.48	21.62
	s	0.97	0.85	1.10	1.16
$C_{18:1}$	$\bar{x}$	47.60 *A*	45.76 *B*	38.60	37.54
	s	1.49	1.23	1.62	1.48
$C_{18:2}$	$\bar{x}$	5.72 *a*	7.12 *b*	6.35 *A*	8.23 *B*
	s	0.83	0.90	0.75	0.62
$C_{18:3}$	$\bar{x}$	0.32 *a*	0.52 *b*	0.48 *a*	1.00 *b*
	s	0.08	0.07	0.08	0.14
$C_{20:0}$	$\bar{x}$	2.14	2.12	1.39	1.41
	s	0.50	0.46	0.35	0.40
$C_{20:1}$	$\bar{x}$	1.44	1.88	0.38	0.40
	s	0.09	0.10	0.09	0.06
$C_{20:2}$	$\bar{x}$	0.46	0.48	0.48	0.66
	s	0.07	0.05	0.07	0.09
$C_{21:0}$	$\bar{x}$	1.53	1.40	1.20	1.47
	s	0.22	0.30	0.40	0.36
$C_{22:0}$	$\bar{x}$	0.47	0.43	0.25	0.30
	s	0.10	0.08	0.06	0.04
Total saturated	$\bar{x}$	42.10 *a*	41.11 *b*	51.61 *a*	49.77 *b*
Total monounsaturated	$\bar{x}$	51.40	50.77	41.08	40.34
Total polyunsaturated	$\bar{x}$	6.50 *A*	8.12 *B*	7.31 *A*	0.89 *B*
Total unsaturated	$\bar{x}$	57.90 *a*	58.89 *b*	48.39 *a*	50.23 *b*

$\bar{x}$ – average value, s – standard deviation
a, b – values with different superscripts are significantly different $P<0.05$
A, B – values with different superscripts are higly significantly different $P<0.01$

low fat level in comparison with back fat and suet of pigs of control group. The back fat of group D had higher ($P<0.05$) coefficient of refraction, a highly statistically significant lower melting point, and higher ($P<0.01$) iodine number than the back fat of pigs of group K. In suet of pigs of group D were ascertained higher ($P<0.05$) coefficient of refraction, lower ($P<0.01$), melting point, and higher ($P<0.05$) iodine number in comparison with group K.

In the amount of fatty acids with shorter chain (C_{10}, C_{12}, C_{14} and C_{15}) in back fat of pigs no statistically significant differences were observed between groups (Table 3). As regards content of acid $C_{16:0}$ there were observed statistically highly significant differences between group K and D. It is interesting to note the statistically significant increase ($P<0.01$) in the amount of acids $C_{17:0}$ and $C_{17:1}$ 1 in the back fat of pigs of group D as compared with control group. A lesser amount ($P<0.05$) of acid $C_{18:0}$ was found in the back fat of group K than of group D. More ($P<0.01$) of acid $C_{18:1}$ had back fat in control group as compared with experimental group. In pigs of group D was observed statistically significant increase of levels of acids $C_{18:2}$ and $C_{18:3}$ in back fat comparing with control group. More ($P<0.05$) of saturated fatty acids were observed in the back fat of pigs of group K than the group D.

A highly statistically significant differences between groups were observed in the amount of total polyunsaturated fatty acids. Statistically significant more of total unsaturated fatty acids were in back fat of group D than the group K.

The suet of pigs of group D contained higher ($P<0.01$) content of acids $C_{17:0}$, $C_{17:1}$ and $C_{18:2}$ than the group K. Statistically significant differences between groups were ascertained in contents of acid $C_{18:3}$. The suet of pigs of group K contained more ($P<0.05$) of total saturated fatty acids and less ($P<0.01$) total polyunsaturated and total unsaturated ($P<0.05$) fatty acids.

4. Discussion

The results of experiments have shown, that the part in complete mixture of krill meal at decreased chitin contents had influence on the physicochemical properties of depot fat in pig fattening.

The research has shown, that the back fat of pigs of control group had higher meling point, lower coefficient of refraction and lower iodine number as compared with the back fat of pigs fed with krill added mixture of decreased chitin contents. The fat of pigs of control group was harder and contained less total unsaturated fatty acids, than the fat of experimental group. The values obtained for physicochemical factors of back fat are similar to the values obtained by other authors (GLAPŚ et al., 1980; MYRES and BOWLAND, 1972). The complete mixtures exerted definite influence on the percent fatty acids content in back fat of fattening pigs. In the back fat of pigs fed with mixtures with krill meal there was observed lesser amount of total saturated fatty acids and increased amount of total unsaturated fatty acids compared with control group. Similar results were obtained by other authors (GLAPŚ et al., 1980; LEWICKI et al., 1977; TAYLOR and THOMKE, 1964), who have used pigs krill meal with all chitin in feeding. In the back fat of pigs there was found an amount of $C_{17:0}$ and $C_{17:1}$. In the fat of pigs of control group was found acid $C_{17:0}$ 0.29 % and $C_{17:1}$ 0.12 % and in the group fed with mixture with krill meal additional was acid $C_{17:0}$ 0.82 % and $C_{17:1}$ 0.59 %.

LEWICKI and al. (1977) in the back fat of pigs fed with mixture containing krill meal with all chitin observed appearance of acid $C_{17:0}$ and $C_{17:1}$ in amount 0.3 % and these acids appeared in trace amounts in back fat of control group. Some authors like VIRTANEN (1967) and MAGIDMAN and al. (1963) have shown, that in natural animal fat there also appear amounts of fatty acids with odd amount carbon atoms in a molecule. One may suppose, that in the research fat of krill meal at decreased chitin contained about 50 % of chitin content when compared with fat of concentrate Provit which contained more fatty acids with odd amount carbon atoms and part of these fatty acids no did not undergo chemical change in organism of pigs but remained and has been built into the fat structure increasing fatty acids content with an odd number of carbons in the chain. The suet of pigs of control group contained greater amount of saturated fatty acids compared with the experimental group. Results obtained for suet fatty acids composition confirmed the data obtained in refraction, melting point and iodine number. The difference in found the degree of saturation of fatty acids of back fat and suet of fattening pigs between groups may have influence on the permanence of the examined fats both in the tissue from and after heating. The obtained results of fatty acids composition of back fat and suet are in agreement with the observations of other authors (GLAPŚ et al., 1980; LEWICKI et al., 1977), who fed pigs with the mixture of krill meal and chitin.

The back fat of fattening pigs fed with mixture including krill meal at lowered chitin to about 50 % contained higher amount of water and less fat in comparison with back fat of control group. Feeding pigs with complete mixture including krill meal at lowered chitin contents resulted in the decreased amount of total saturated fatty acids and increased amount of total unsaturated fatty acids in back fat and suet. Back fat and suet of pigs fed with mixture including krill meal will be less permanent than the back fat and suet of pigs of control group. Feeding pigs with complete mixture including krill meal at lowered chitin content to about 50 % resulted in the deterioration of quality back fat and suet.

Summary

The aim of this research was to determine the impact of feeding fattening pigs with krill meal added mixture at lowered chitin content to about 50 % on the physiochemical properties of depot fat.

The obtained results show, that feeding pigs with complete mixture with krill meal added at lowered chitin content resulted in the decreased amount of saturated fatty acids and increased amount of unsaturated fatty acids in back fat and suet.

Zusammenfassung

MARIA KREŁOWSKA-KUŁAS

Der Einfluß des Krillmehlanteils mit vermindertem Chitingehalt im Mischfutter für Mastschweine auf die Qualität des Reservefettes

Die Untersuchungen wurden am Fettgewebe von in zwei Gruppen eingeteilten Mastschweinen durchgeführt. Es sollte den Einfluß der Fütterung von Mastschweinen mit einem Krillmehl enthaltenden Mischfutter auf die physikalisch-chemischen Eigenschaften des Reservefettes bestimmen. Das verwendete Krillmehl enthielt einen um 50 % verminderten Chitingehalt. Die gewonnenen Ergebnisse zeigen, daß die Fütterung der Mastschweine mit der Krillmehl-Ration eine Verminderung der Menge an gesättigten Fettsäuren und eine Erhöhung der Menge an ungesättigten Fettsäuren in Speck und Fett bewirkt.

Резюме

Мария Креловска-Кулас

Влияние частоты крыляной муки с пониженным содержанием в смеси хитина для откормочников на качество запасного жира

Исследование проведено на жировой ткани 60 свиней разделённых на две группы. Целью исследований было определение влияния откорма откормочников смесью с добавлением муки из крыля с пониженным на 50 % содержанием хитина, на физико-химинеские особенности запасного жира.

Полученные результаты указывают, что откорм свиней полноценной смесью с добавлением муки из крыля с пониженным содержанием хитина повлияло на уменьшение количества насыщенных жирных кислот и увеличение количества ненасыщенных кислот в шпиге и свином сале.

References

[1] BLIGH, E. G., and W. J. DYER: Can. J. Biochem. Physiol. **37**, 911 (1959)
[2] ENDRESS, J. G.: J. Am. Oil Chem. Soc. **43**, 600 (1966)
[3] GLAPŚ, J., A. KORNIEWICZ and E. BOROWA: Rocz. Nauk. Zoot., Monografie i rozprawy, **16**, 37 (1980)
[4] KOTARBIŃSKA, M., and K. GROSZYK: Nowe Rol. **6**, 27 (1977)
[5] LEAT, W. M. T., A. CUTHBERSTON, A. W. HOWARD and G. A. GRESHAM: J. agricult. Sci. Camb. **63**, 311 (1964)
[6] LEWICKI, C., J. TYWOŃCZUK and T. RAKOWSKA: MASZYNOPIS ART Olsztyn (1977)
[7] MAGIDMAN, P., S. F. HART, F. E. LUDDER and R. W. REIMENSCHNEIDER: J. Anim. Oil Chemistry Soc. **40**, 86 (1963)
[8] MYRES, A. W., and J. P. BOWLAND: Can. J. Anim. Sci. **52**, 113 (1972)
[9] PASTUSZEWSKA, B.: Post. Nauk Roln. **4**, 59 (1979)
[10] PEZACKI, W., Z. DUDA and G. WASILEWICZ: Gosp. Mięsna, **7**, 1 (1967)
[11] RUTKOWSKI, A., and K. KRYGIER: Technologia i analiza tłuszczów jadalnych, SGGW Warszawa (1979)
[12] RUSZCZYC, Z.: Metodyka doświadczeń zootechnicznych, PWRiL, Warszawa (1978).
[13] TAYLOR, M., and S. THOMKE: Nature, **201**, 1246 (1964)
[14] VIRTANEN, N. J.: Urea and protein supplement H. Briggs, Pergamon Press, 185 (1967)

Received: 1 October 1986

Address of author:

Doc. dr. habil. MARIA KREŁOWSKA-KUŁAS,
Institute of Commodity Science,
Academy of Economics,
Sienkiewicza 4,
30–033 Kraków,
Poland

Arch. Anim. Nutr., Berlin 37 (1987) 6, 539–548

Sektion Tierproduktion und Veterinärmedizin der Karl-Marx Universität Leipzig, Wissenschaftsbereich Tierernährungsphysiologie und Futtermittelkunde (Leiter: Prof. Dr. sc. G. GEBHARDT)[1])
LPG (P) „Paul Fröhlich“ Leipzig (Vors.: Dr. A. SCHWEIGEL)[2])
Sektion Pflanzenproduktion der Martin-Luther-Universität Halle-Wittenberg, Lehrstuhl Ackerfutter (Leiter: Prof. Dr. sc. B. MÀRTIN)[3])

SIGRUN SOUFFRANT[2], H. JEROCH[1] und W. RÖTSCKE[3]

Futterwert von Grünmais in Hauptfruchtstellung

1. Einleitung

Grünmais zählt zu den ertragreichsten Grünfutterpflanzen (GEORG, 1984; RÖTSCHKE und JEROCH, 1986; SIMON und WEILAND, 1984), dessen Bedeutung als stabile Komponente in der Frischfutterversorgung der Rinder von Ende Juli bis Mitte Oktober in zunehmendem Maße von den Landwirtschaftsbetrieben erkannt wird. In der Jungbullenmast ermöglicht der Einsatz von Grünmais als alleiniges Grobfutter in Verbindung mit einem proteinreichen Ergänzungsfutter (konzentratarmer Rationstyp) hohe Zunahmen (JEROCH u. a., 1984; SOUFFRANT und WYRWICH, 1985).

Die Angaben zum Futterwert von Grünmais sind jedoch sehr lückenhaft. Im DDR-Futterbewertungssystem (AUTORENKOLLEKTIV, 1977) wird Grünmais nicht gesondert ausgewiesen. Nach Angaben von POPOW (1963) sowie STÄHLIN und CRÖSSMANN (1968) nimmt die Verdaulichkeit der Rohnährstoffe von Grünmais im Verlauf der Vegetation ab. In Fütterungsversuchen mit Mastbullen (GEORG, 1984; JEROCH u. a., 1984) wurde demgegenüber kein Rückgang der Futterqualität festgestellt. Eine systematische Untersuchung des Futterwertes von Grünmais erwies sich deshalb als notwendig. Neben der Erfassung des Ertragsverlaufes von Grünmais, der als Hauptfrucht, zeitige und späte Zweitfrucht angebaut wurde und deren jeweilige Nutzungsspanne sich über den bisher empfohlenen Zeitraum von 20 bis 25 Tagen erstreckte, sollten vor allem der Nährstcffgehalt, die Verdaulichkeit sowie die Energie- und Proteinkonzentration von Grünmais über eine relativ lange Vegetationszeit ermittelt werden. Vorliegender Beitrag berichtet über die in 4jährigen Untersuchungen erhaltenen Ergebnisse von Grünmais in Hauptfruchtstellung.

2. Material und Methoden

2.1. Feldversuche

In den Jahren 1982 bis 1985 wurden auf Produktionsschlägen der LPG Pflanzenproduktion „Paul Fröhlich“ Leipzig kontinuierliche Feldversuche durchgeführt. Dazu wurde Grünmais zu drei Saatzeiten gelegt und zwar in Hauptfruchtstellung (Saat bis 5. 5.), als frühe Zweitfrucht (Saat bis 25. 5.) und späte Zweitfrucht (Saat bis 15. 6.). Beginnend mit dem Entwicklungsstadium „Beginn der Blüte“ wurde täglich die benötigte Frischfuttermenge für die Verdauungsversuche als Ganzpflanze mittels Sichel bzw. mit einem Mähbinder (1985) geerntet und Erntefläche sowie Frischmasseertrag ermittelt. Außerdem erfolgte die Erfassung von Wuchshöhe und Bestandesdichte (Pflanzen/m^2). In Tabelle 1 sind einige wichtige agrotechnische Daten des ersten Saattermines (Hauptfrucht) der vier Untersuchungsjahre zusammengestellt.

Tabelle 1 (Table 1)
Agrotechnische Daten der Grünmaisversuche
(Agricultural dates of the experiment with green maize)

Jahr (Year)	Sorte (Sort)	Aussaattermin (Sowing time)	Bestandsdichte (Pfl./ha) (Plant density, plant/ha)	Prüfzeitraum (Test periode) Datum (Date)	Vegetationstage (Growth days)	Erntetage (Harvest days)
1982	BEKOS 251	30. 4. 82	227000	19. 7.–10. 9.	80–134	54
1983	BEKE 246	5. 5. 83	226500	22. 7.–21. 9.	78–140	62
1984	BEKE 246	28. 4. 84	216000	6. 8.–17. 10.	100–172	72
1985	BEKE 246	25. 4. 85	190700	31. 7.– 8. 10.	97–166	69

Nach Zerkleinerung der Maispflanzen (Häcksellänge 20 bis 40 mm) erfolgte täglich die Futterprobenahme für die Nährstoffanalyse, wobei entsprechend der Versuchsgestaltung jeweils fünf Teilproben zu einer Sammelprobe vereinigt wurden (5 Tage = 1 Versuchsperiode).

2.2. Tierversuche

Die Ermittlung der Verdaulichkeit der Rohnährstoffe des Grünmaises erfolgte nach dem kontinuierlichen Verfahren an vier ausgewachsenen Hammeln der Rasse Merinofleischschaf. Grundlage für die Gestaltung der Verdauungsversuche bildeten die methodischen Richtlinien zur Durchführung von Verdauungsversuchen für die Futterwertschätzung (SCHIEMANN, 1981). Die Tiere wurden einzeln in Stoffwechselkäfigen mit Harnabfluß gehalten. Der gehäckselte Grünmais kam als Alleinfutter zum Einsatz. Zur Deckung des Vitamin-, Mineralstoff- und Rohproteinbedarfs wurden das Vitaminpräparat „Mileipan", die Mineralstoffmischung für Rinder mit 133 g Phosphor pro kg und Harnstoff verabreicht. Tränkwasser stand den Tieren ad libitum zur Verfügung. Die Sammlung des Kotes erfolgte mittels Kotbeutel. In der Hauptperiode wurde täglich zur Morgenfütterung die Kotmenge erfaßt, eine aliquote Menge entnommen, zur Sammelprobe vereinigt und bis zur Aufbereitung im gefrorenen Zustand gelagert. Dabei wurde die Kotsammelperiode gegenüber der Fütterungsperiode um drei Tage verschoben.

2.3. Analytische Untersuchungen

Die chemisch-analytischen Untersuchungen der Futter- und Kotproben umfaßte die Bestimmung des Trockensubstanzgehaltes sowie die Rohnährstoffzusammensetzung nach dem Weender-Verfahren. Die Rohfettbestimmung erfolgte nach vorherigem

HCl-Aufschluß. 1982 und 1983 wurden die Futterproben hinsichtlich ihres Stärke- und Zuckergehaltes untersucht.*

Die Untersuchungen wurden nach modifizierten Arbeitsvorschriften durchgeführt; für die Stärke in Anlehnung an CLEGG (1956) und HEHL (1973) und für Zucker (Glukose-Äquivalent) in Anlehnung an KLUSAK (1977).

2.4. Auswertung

Die Auswertung des umfangreichen Datenmaterials erfolgte regressionsanalytisch. Zur Anwendung kamen das lineare (y = a + bx) und das quadratische ($y = a + bx + cx^2$) Modell der Regressionsanalyse. Für die zusammenfassende Darstellung der vier Untersuchungsjahre wurde der Trockensubstanzgehalt der Maisganzpflanze als geeignete Bezugsbasis gewählt. Auf der Grundlage des ermittelten Trockensubstanzgehaltes des Grünmaises wurden die Veränderungen des Rohnährstoffgehaltes und der Verdaulichkeit der Rohnährstoffe regressiv verrechnet. Die analysierten Rohnährstoffe und die am Schaf gemessene scheinbare Verdaulichkeit dienten der Berechnung der Gehalte an Energetischen Futtereinheiten – Rind (EFr) und verdaulichem Rohprotein (vRP). Die Auswertung erfolgte im Trockensubstanzbereich von 13 bis 25 %.

3. Ergebnisse und Diskussion

In diesem Beitrag werden die Ergebnisse des ersten Saattermines (Hauptfruchtstellung ≙ Saat bis 5. Mai) vorgestellt. In einer späteren Mitteilung ist die Auswertung der zweiten (frühe Zweitfrucht) und dritten (späte Zweitfrucht) Saatzeit vorgesehen.

3.1. Ertragsentwicklung

Grünmais gilt als erntewürdig, wenn die Fahne (männliche Blüte) erscheint (LÜDDECKE, 1976; STÄHLIN und CRÖSSMANN, 1968). Zu diesem Zeitpunkt befindet sich der Pflanzenbestand noch in der Phase der Sproßstreckung und Blattausbildung und

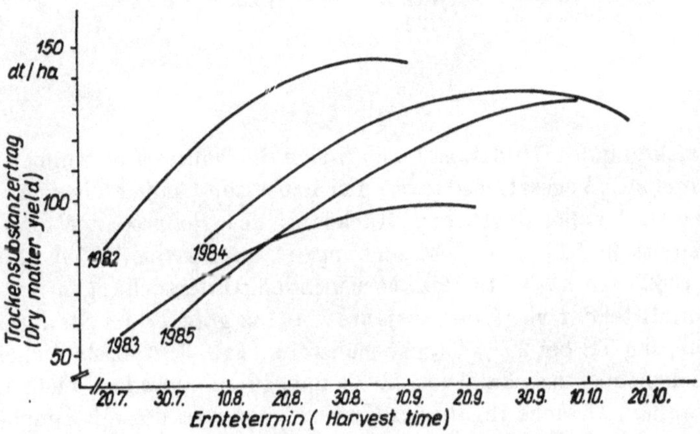

Abb. 1 (Fig. 1). Entwicklung des Trockensubstanzertrages von Grünmais in Abhängigkeit vom Erntetermin (Development of the dry matter yield of green maize in dependence on the harvest time).

* Herrn Dr. SCHLEGELMILCH vom Zentrallabor der Martin-Luther-Universität Halle, Sektion Pflanzenproduktion, sei an dieser Stelle für die Übernahme und Durchführung der Analysen gedankt.

somit in einer Etappe hohen Ertragszuwachses. In dieser Entwicklungsphase – bis etwa zur beginnenden Milchreife im Korn – bringt Grünmais mit seinen dichteren Beständen höhrere Erträge als Silomais (BROUWER, 1972; KREIL u. a., 1983; SIMON und WEILAND, 1984). So sind bereits in der letzten Julidekade, in Abhängigkeit von der Witterung, Trockensubstanzerträge von 60 ... 100 dt/ha erreichbar, die im Verlauf der Vegetation noch weiter ansteigen. Die Entwicklung des Trockensubstanzertrages in Abhängigkeit vom Erntetermin in den einzelnen Untersuchungsjahren ist in Abbildung 1 dargestellt. Diese Darstellung vermittelt einen deutlichen Einfluß der Witterung auf das Ertragsniveau. Die Sommertrockenheit 1982 führte zu einem hohen Ertrag bereits zu Beginn der Ernteperiode und der weiter ansteigende Trockensubstanzgehalt hatte bei den späteren Ernten noch beträchtliche Steigerungen des Ertrages an Trockensubstanz zur Folge. Die feucht-kühle Witterung während der Jugendentwicklung im Jahre 1984 bewirkte einen späteren Nutzungsbeginnn aber noch einen erheblichen Ertragszuwachs während der Nutzungszeit. Dennoch konnten auch zu Versuchsende nicht ähnlich hohe Trockensubstanzgehalte wie in den anderen Versuchsjahren erreicht werden (Tab. 2).

Tabelle 2 (Table 2)

Trockensubstanzerträge und Trockensubstanzgehalte von Grünmais zu Beginn und am Ende der Nutzungszeitspanne (Dry matter yield and dry matter content of green maize at the beginning and at the end of the period of utilization)

Jahr (Year)	Nutzungszeitspanne (Tage nach der Saat) (Period of utilization; days after sowing)	Trockensubstanzertrag (dt/ha) (Dry matter yield [dt/ha]) Nutzungsbeginn (Beginning of utilization)	Nutzungsende (End of utilization)	Trockensubstanzgehalt %) (Dry matter content [%]) Nutzungsbeginn (Beginning of utilization	Nutzungsende End of utilization
1982	80 ... 134	88	146	14,3	27,6
1983	78 ... 140	57	83	15.0	28,1
1984	100 ... 172	100	134	13.3	23,3
1985	97 ... 166	59	132	16,1	28,6

3.2. Nährstoffgehalt

Mit fortschreitender Entwicklung des Grünmaises ändert sich die Nährstoffzusammensetzung (Tab. 3). Zunehmende Vegetationsdauer, gleichzusetzen mit steigendem Trockensubstanzgehalt, bewirkt einen deutlichen Rückgang des *Rohproteingehaltes*. Dieses Resultat wurde bereits in früheren Untersuchungen von DAWLA (1978) und RÖTSCHKE und GEORG (1982) ermittelt. In den vorliegenden Untersuchungen verringerte sich der Gehalt im Mittel der vier Versuchsjahre von 132 g/kg TS im Stadium „Beginn der Blüte" auf 90 g/kg TS bei 25 % Trockensubstanz (Tab. 3, Abb. 2), wobei die Werte ab einem Trockensubstanzgehalt von 20 % nahezu unverändert bleiben und um 90 g/kg TS schwanken. Ursache für diesen Kurvenverlauf ist der mit zunehmendem Alter der Pflanze rückläufige Rohproteingehalt in den Blättern und Stengeln, während der sich bildende Kolben mit seinem steigenden Proteingehalt einen weiteren Abfall kompensiert (BROUWER, 1972).

Tabelle 3 (Table 3)

Entwicklung der Rohnährstoffzusammensetzung, der Verdaulichkeit der organischen Substanz und der Energie sowie der Energie- und Proteinkonzentration von Grünmais in Abhängigkeit vom Trockensubstanzgehalt (Development of crude nutrients, of digestibility of the organic matter and of the energy, the energy- and protein concentration in dependence on dry matter content)

Trockensubstanzgehalt (%) (Dry matter content [%])	Rohnährstoffgehalt (g/kg TS) (Crude nutrients content, g/kg DM)				Verdaulichkeit (%) (Digestibility [%])		Energiekonzentration[1] (Energy concentration)	Proteinkonzentration[2] (Protein concentration)
	Rohprotein- (Crude protein)	Rohfaser (Crude fibre)	N-freie Extraktstoffe (N-free extractives)	Stärke (Starch)	org. Substanz (Organic matter)	Energie (Energy)		
13	132	278	482	19	69	66	525	76
15	118	258	528	10	71	68	542	72
17	106	242	566	9	72	69	555	68
19	98	228	596	16	73	69	565	64
21	92	218	618	33	73	70	569	60
23	89	211	631	58	73	69	570	56
25	90	206	634	93	72	68	568	52

1) Energetische Futtereinheiten – Rind/kg Trockensubstanz (Energetic feed unit–cattle/kg dry matter

2) g verdauliches Rohprotein/kg Trockensubstanz (g digestible crude protein/kg dry matter)

Grünmais unterscheidet sich von anderen Futterpflanzen durch den mit fortschreitender Vegetation sinkenden *Rohfasergehalt* (Tab. 3, Abb. 3). Nach Abschluß des intensiven Längenwachstums nimmt der Rohfaseranteil im Stengel nicht weiter zu. Eine Verschiebung innerhalb der Kohlenhydratfraktion, bedingt durch die verstärkte Zuckereinlagerung, führt zu einem Rückgang des Rohfasergehaltes im Stengel (Brouwer, 1972). Die mangelhafte Kolbenausbildung dichter Grünmaisbestände bewirkt, daß die Blätter einen größeren Anteil an der Gesamtpflanze ausmachen als beim Silomais. Daraus resultiert der etwas höhere Rohfasergehalt des Grünmaises gegenüber Silomais.

In den vorliegenden Untersuchungen verminderte sich der Gehalt an Gerüstkohlenhydraten von 278 g/kg TS auf 206 g/kg TS. Innerhalb des Rohfaserkomplexes übt der Ligningehalt einen deutlichen Einfluß auf die Verdaulichkeit aus. Nach Brouwer (1972) bleibt der Ligningehalt beim Mais, im Gegensatz zu anderen Ge-

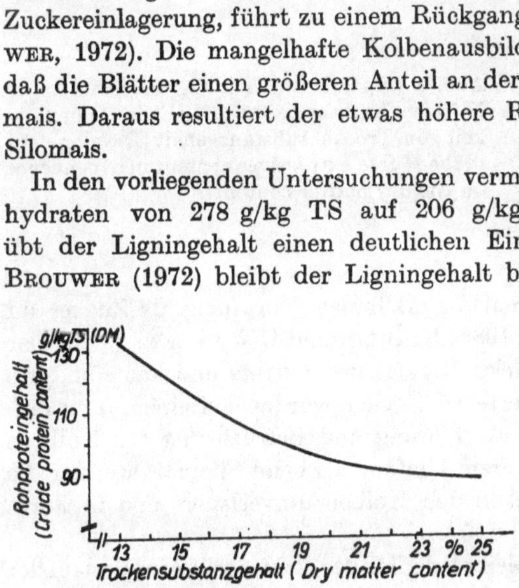

Abb. 2 (Fig. 2). Entwicklung des Rohproteingehaltes in Abhängigkeit vom Trockensubstanzgehalt (Development of the crude protein content in dependence on the dry matter content).

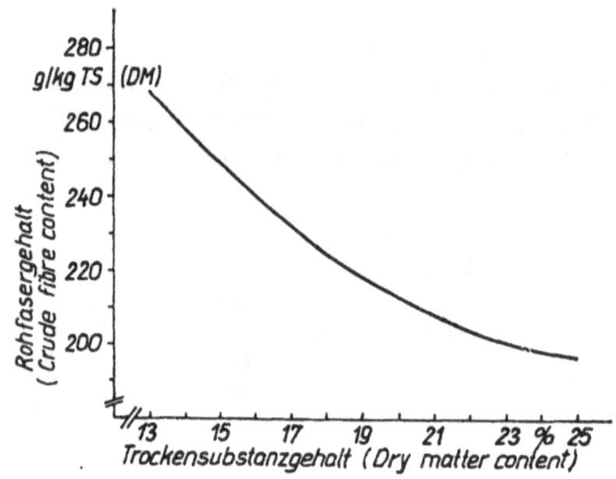

Abb. 3 (Fig. 3). Entwicklung des Rohfasergehaltes in Abhängigkeit vom Trockensubstanzgehalt (Development of the crude fibre content in dependence on the dry matter content).

treidearten, von der Vollblüte bis zur Milchreife etwa gleich und nimmt erst danach wieder zu. Außerdem weisen dichtere Bestände einen um etwa 1% niedrigeren Ligningehalt als lockere Bestände auf. Die größten Veränderungen vollziehen sich in der Fraktion der *N-freien Extraktstoffe* (NFE). Der Gehalt an NFE nimmt im Laufe der Vegetation deutlich zu (Tab. 3, Abb. 4). Bis zu einem Trockensubstanzgehalt von 20 % ist ein steiler Anstieg der NFE-Fraktion (von 482 g/kg TS auf 608 g/kg TS) zu beobachten, während der Kurvenverlauf danach deutlich abflacht. Bei weiter ansteigendem Trockensubstanzgehalt (über 25 %) deutet sich eine leicht rückläufige Tendenz an. Die Zusammensetzung der NFE-Fraktion unterliegt im Verlauf der physiologischen Entwicklung des Maises ebenfalls beachtlichen Veränderungen. Bei Grünmais mit meist

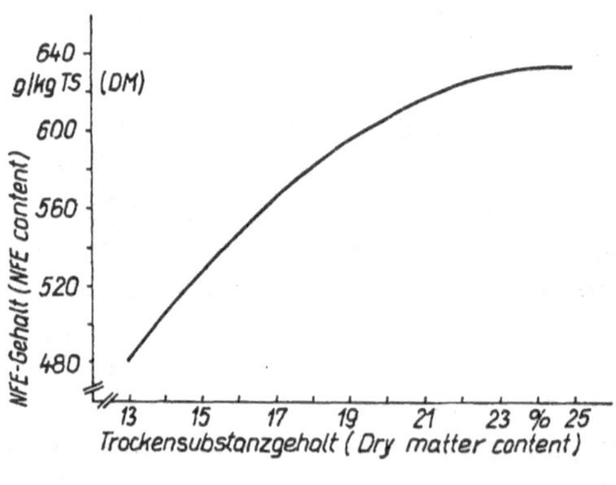

Abb. 4 (Fig. 4). Entwicklung des Gehaltes an N-freien Extraktstoffen (NFE) in Abhängigkeit vom Trockensubstanzgehalt (Development of the N-free extractives content in dependence on the dry matter content).

nur mangelhafter Kolbenausbildung werden die Assimilate vorrangig als Zucker im Stengel abgelagert (SIMON und WEILAND, 1984; STÄHLIN und CRÖSSMANN, 1968). Der hohe Zuckergehalt begünstigt die Schmackhaftigkeit des Futters und hat eine gute Futteraufnahme zur Folge. Die Höchstwerte an Zucker wurden bei einem Trockensubstanzgehalt von 21 % ermittelt. Nach Ausbildung und Befruchtung des Kolbens setzt die Kornfüllungsphase ein. In geringerem Umfang als beim Silomais werden die löslichen Kohlenhydrate aus dem Stengel in den Kolben umverlagert und in Form von Stärke in den Körnern gespeichert (Abb. 5.).

Von den einzelnen Nährstoffgruppen bleibt lediglich der *Rohfettgehalt* im Verlauf der Vegetation weitgehend konstant. Die Werte liegen im Bereich von 16 bis 19 g/kg TS.

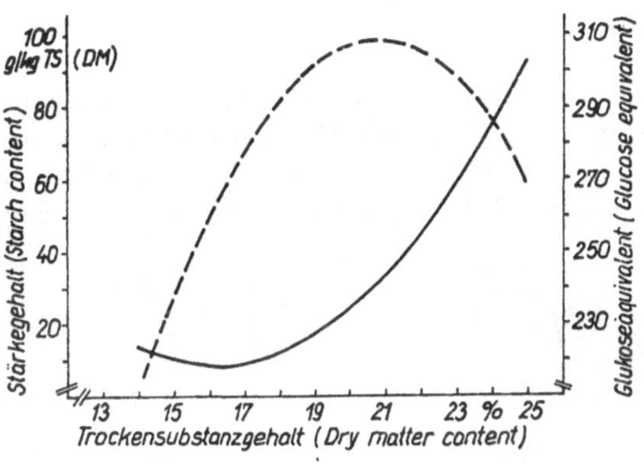

Abb. 5 (Fig. 5). Entwicklung des Glukoseäquivalentes und des Stärkegehaltes in Abhängigkeit vom Trockensubstanzgehalt (Development of the glucose equivalent and the starch content in dependence on the dry matter content).

- - - - - - Glukoseäquivalent (Glucose equivalent)

——— Stärkegehalt (Content of starch).

3.3. Verdaulichkeit der Rohnährstoffe, der organischen Substanz und der Energie

Die Auswertung der durchgeführten Verdauungsversuche ergab, daß die Verdaulichkeit der einzelnen Rohnährstoffe (Abb. 6) über einen relativ langen Vegetationszeitraum nur geringen, die Verdaulichkeit der organischen Substanz und der Energie nur

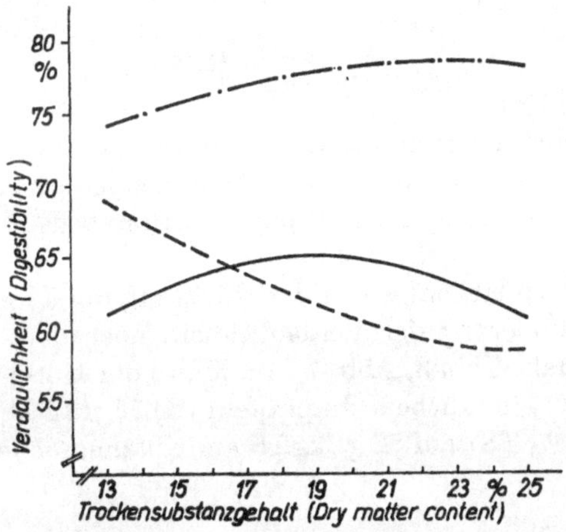

Abb. 6 (Fig. 6). Verdaulichkeit der Rohnährstoffe (Rohprotein, Rohfaser, N-freie Extraktstoffe) in Abhängigkeit vom Trockensubstanzgehalt (Digestibility of nutrients (crude protein, crude fibre, N-free extractives) in dependence on the dry matter content).

—·—·— N-freie Extraktstoffe (N-free extractives)

——— Rohfaser (Crude fibre)

- - - - - - Rohprotein (Crude protein).

unbedeutenden Veränderungen unterliegt. Am deutlichsten ist der Abfall der Rohproteinverdaulichkeit um 11 Einheiten von 69 % auf 58 %. Die Rohfaserverdaulichkeit zeigt keine eindeutige Beziehung zu den Veränderungen der Gehaltswerte. Trotz beachtlichem Rückgang der Rohfaserfraktion variiert die Verdaulichkeit nur um 4 Einheiten zwischen 61 und 65 % und zeigt erst ab $>$ 21 % Trockensubstanz eine abnehmende Tendenz. Diese Aussage bestätigt, daß erst mit weiter steigendem Trockensubstanzgehalt die Verdaulichkeit der Rohfaserfraktion, infolge Anstieg des Ligninanteils, negativ beeinflußt wird. Die Verdaulichkeit der N-freien Extraktstoffe unterliegt ebenfalls nur geringfügigen Veränderungen (4 Einheiten) und bleibt ab $\geqq$ 17 % Trockensubstanz mit 77 – 78 % nahezu konstant.

Die Verdaulichkeit organischer Substanz und Energie verändert sich im untersuchten Trockensubstanzbereich von 13 bis 25 %, also über einen relativ langen Nutzungszeitraum, kaum (Tab. 3); sie beträgt für die organische Substanz 72 % bzw. für die Energie 69 %.

3.4. Energie- und Proteinkonzentration

Über die Veränderung der Energiekonzentration mit fortschreitender Vegetation im Mittel der Untersuchungsjahre informieren Tab. 3 und Abb. 7. Deutlich wird der steile Anstieg der Energikonzentration von 525 bei 13 % Trockensubstanz auf 560 bei 18 %, während die Veränderungen danach wesentlich langsamer verlaufen und zwischen

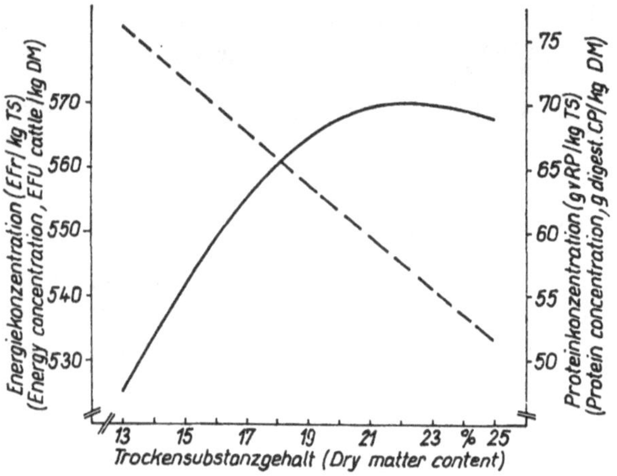

Abb. 7 (Fig. 7). Entwicklung der Energie- und Rohproteinkonzentration in Abhängigkeit vom Trockensubstanzgehalt (Development of energy- and crude protein content in dependence on the dry matter content).

560 und 570 EFr/kg TS schwanken. Grünmais liefert somit über einen relativ langen Erntezeitraum ein Grobfutter mit nahezu gleichbleibendem hohen energetischen Futterwert, was für die praktische Rationsgestaltung in der Rinderfütterung bedeutsam ist.

Mais zählt zu den proteinarmen Grünfutterpflanzen, wobei der Rückgang der Proteinkonzentration, bedingt durch die Verminderung der Verdaulichkeit, noch deutlicher ausgeprägt ist als beim Rohproteingehalt (Tab. 3, Abb. 7). Im Mittel der Untersuchungsjahre verringerte sich der Gehalt an verdaulichem Rohprotein von 76g/kg TS zu Beginn des Untersuchungszeitraumes (13 % TS) auf 52 g//kg TS am Nutzungsende (25 % TS).

Zusammenfassung

Zur Erweiterung der Kenntnisse über den Futterwert von Grünmais im Verlauf der Vegetation wurden in den Jahren 1982 bis 1985 Feldversuche mit Grünmais, angebaut in Hauptfruchtstellung (Saat bis 5. 5.), durchgeführt. Das dabei gewonnene Erntegut wurde in kontinuierlichen Verdauungsversuchen geprüft.

Die Auswertung der durchgeführten Untersuchungen umfaßt den Trockensubstanzbereich von 13 bis 25 %. In diesem Bereich vermindert sich der Rohproteingehalt von 132 auf 90 g/kg TS und der Rohfasergehalt von 278 auf 206 g/kg TS. Der Gehalt an N-freien Extraktstoffen steigt von 482 auf 634 g/kg TS an. Lediglich der Rohfettgehalt bleibt mit Werten zwischen 16 und 19 g/kg TS weitgehend unverändert.

Die Verdaulichkeit der einzelnen Rohährstoffe weist mit Ausnahme des Rohproteins nur geringe Veränderungen auf (Rohfaserverdaulichkeit 61 bis 65 %; NFE-Verdaulichkeit 74 bis 78 %; Rohproteinverdaulichkeit 69 → 58 %). Nahezu konstant bleiben die

Verdaulichkeiten von organischer Substanz (72 %) und Energie (69 %). Bis zu 18 % Trockensubstanz nimmt die Energiekonzentration deutlich zu; danach besitzt Grünmais einen energetischen Futterwert von 560 bis 570 Energetischen Futtereinheiten-Rind/kg TS. Die Proteinkonzentration (g verdauliches Rohprotein/kg TS) verringert sich im untersuchten Trockensubstanzbereich der Pflanze von 76 auf 52 g/kg TS.

Резюме

Зигрун Зоуффрант, Х. Ерох и В. Рётшке

Питательность кукурузы на зелёный корм как главной культуры

В процессе изучения питательности кукурузы на зелёный корм во время вегетации проводилось в гг. 1982–1985 возделивание кукурузы на зелёный корм как главной культуры на опытном поле, т. е. 5. 5. последний срок посева. Полученный урожай исследовался в постоянных переваримых опытах.

Сообщаются результаты исследования в пределах от 13 по 25 % сухого вещества. Здесь уменьшается содержание сырого протеина от 132 до 90 г/кг сухого в-ва, а для клетчатки определилось снижение от 278 до 206 г/кг сухого в-ва. Содержание БЭВа повышается от 482 до 634 г/кг сухого в-ва. Только относительно содержания сырого жира почти нет изменения, данные колебаются от 16 до 19г / кг сухого в-ва.

Переваримость отдельных сырых питательных веществ с исключением сырого протеина почти не изменяется (переваримость клетчатки от 61 до 65 %, переваримость БЭВа от 74 до 78 %, переваримость сырого протеина снижается от 69 до 58 %.) Тоже не изменились переваримости органического вещества (72 %) и энергии (69 %). До содержания сухого вещества от 18 % концентрация энергии значительно повышается, т. е. кукуруза на зелёный корм содержит от 560 до 570 $ЭКЕ_{крс}$/кг сухого в-ва. Концентрация протеина в г переваримого сырого протеина/кг сухого в-ва снижается в исследуемых пределах содержания сухого вещества растения от 76 до 52 г/кг сухого в-ва.

Summary

Sigrun Souffrant, H. Jeroch and W. Rötschke

Feed value of green maize as main crop

In order to extend the knowledge of the feed value of green maize in the course of vegetation, field experiments with green maize as main crop (seed time before May 5) were carried out between 1982 and 1985. The crop thus yielded was tested in continuous digestion experiments.

The assessment of this study comprises a dry matter range of between 13 and 25 %. In this range the crude protein content decreases from 132 to 90 g/kg DM and the crude fibre content from 278 to 206 g/kg DM. The content of N-free extractives increases from 482 to 634 g/kg DM. Only the crude fat content with values between 16 and 19 g/kg DM remains largely unchanged.

The digestibility of the individual crude nutrients, with the exception of crude protein, shows small changes only (digestibility of crude fibre 61–65 %, NfE digestibility 74–78 %, digestibility of crude protein 69–58 %). The digestibility of organic matter (72 %) and energy (69 %) remains nearly constant.

Up to 18 % dry matter the energy concentration increase distinctly; the green maize has an energetic feed value of 560–570 energetic feed units$_{cattle}$/kg DM. The protein concentration (g digestible crude protein/kg DM) in the dry matter range of the plants studied decreased from 76 to 52 g/kg DM.

Literaturverzeichnis

[1] AUTORENKOLLEKTIV: Das DDR-Futterbewertungssystem. 4. unveränd. Aufl. VEB Deutscher Landwirtschaftsverlag Berlin (1977)
[2] BROUWER, W.: Handbuch des speziellen Pflanzenbaues. Paul Parey Verlag, Berlin u. Hamburg (1972)
[3] CLEGG, K. M.: J. Sci. Food Agric. 7, 41 (1956)
[4] DAWLA, N.: Einfluß mehrerer Intensivierungsfaktoren auf den Ertrag und Futterwert von Grünmais. Diss. (Prom. A), Martin-Luther-Univ. Halle – Wittenberg (1978)
[5] GEORG, R.: Einfluß pflanzenbaulicher Maßnahmen auf Ertrag und Qualität bei der Grünmaisproduktion. Diss. (Prom. A), Martin-Luther-Univ. Halle – Wittenberg (1984)
[6] HEHL, G.: Z. Anal. Chem. 266 (1973)
[7] JEROCH, H., G. GEBHARDT, W. RÖTSCHKE, B. MÄRTIN, S. SOUFFRANT und R. ACKERMANN: Tierzucht **38**, 363 (1984)
[8] KLUSAK, H.: Rostlinna, Vyroba, Praha 23 (1977)
[9] KREIL, W., W. SIMON und E. WOJAHN: Futterpflanzenbau-Empfehlungen, Richtwerte, Normative. VEB Deutscher Landwirtschaftsverlag Berlin (1983)
[10] LÜDDECKE, F.: Ackerfutter. VEB Deutscher Landwirtschaftsverlag Berlin (1976)
[11] POPOW, G.: Zum Anbau von Grünmais. Mitt. schweiz. Landwirtschaft **10**, 3 (1963)
[12] RÖTSCHKE, W. und R. GEORG: Der Anbau von Grünmais – ein Beitrag zur Verbesserung der Frischfutterversorgung der Rinderbestände. Tagungsbericht der Akademie der Landwirtschaftswissenschaften der DDR, Nr. 199, Berlin (1982)
[13] RÖTSCHKE, W. und H. JEROCH: Grünmaisanbau und Einsatz in der Fütterung. agra-Buch, Landwirtschaftsausstellung der DDR (1986)
[14] SCHIEMANN, R.: Arch. Tierernähr. **31**, 1 (1981)
[15] SIMON, W. und G. WEILAND: Feldwirtschaft **25**, 72 (1984)
[16] SOUFFRANT, S. und A. WYRWICH: Futterwert und Einsatz von Grünmais in der Bullenmast. Tag.-Ber. 4. Maiskolloquium d. Sekt. Tierprod. u. Vet.med. der Karl-Marx-Univ. Leipzig (1985)
[17] STÄHLIN, A. und G. CRÖSSMANN: Mais als Grünfutterpflanze. Das wirtschaftseigene Futter. Frankfurt/M. **14**, 2 (1968)

Anschrift der Autoren:

Dipl.-Agr.-Ing. SIGRUN SOUFFRANT und Doz. Dr. sc. H. JEROCH
Sektion Tierproduktion und Veterinärmedizin der Karl-Marx-Universität Leipzig,
Wissenschaftsbereich Tierernährungsphysiologie und Futtermittelkunde
Gustav-Kühn-Str. 8
Leipzig
7022 - DDR

Dr. W. RÖTSCHKE
Sektion Pflanzenproduktion der Martin-Luther-Universität Halle – Wittenberg,
Lehrstuhl Ackerfutter
Emil-Abderhalden-Str. 25
Halle (Saale)
4010 - DDR

Arch. Anim. Nutr., Berlin 37 (1987) 6, 549–550

Buchbesprechungen

Umweltvorschriften für die Landwirtschaft. Verfasser: Dr. HANS-JOACHIM HÖTZEL. Erschienen im Verlag Eugen Ulmer Stuttgart, 1986; 467 Seiten, Kunststoffeinband, Format 13×20 cm – Preis: DM 58,–

Der Autor Dr. HANS-JOACHIM HÖTZEL ist leitender Landwirtschaftsdirektor in Bonn. Er unterteilt sein Buch zunächst in A „*Allgemeines Agrarumweltrecht*“, B „*Besonderes Agrarumweltrecht*“ und C „*Möglichkeiten und Grenzen der Landwirtschaft nach dem Agrarumweltrecht*“. Dabei umfaßt Kapitel C den Hauptanteil des Buches und unterteilt sich in folgende Unterkapitel: „*Erwerb und Veräußerung von Betrieben und Grundstücken, Pacht und Zupacht*“, „*Flurbereinigung*“, „*Bauen*“, „*Wasserversorgung und Abwasserbeseitigung*“, „*Nutztierhaltung*“, „*Umweltschutz in der Innenwirtschaft*“, „*Nutzungsbeschränkungen nach dem Naturschutz- und Landschaftspflegerecht*“, „*Nutzungsbeschränkungen nach dem Forstrecht*“, „*Bestellungs- und Pflegearbeiten*“, „*Bewässerung, Entwässerung und Gewässerunterhaltung*“, „*Düngung*“, „*Pflanzenschutz*“, „*Erntearbeiten*“ und als 14. Kapitel „*Dienstleistung und Direktvermarktung*“.

Alle gesetzlichen Angaben beziehen sich selbstverständlich auf die Belange der BRD.

Im Kapitel *Nutztierhaltung* werden folgende Unterkapitel ausführlich behandelt: Tierschutz, Fütterung, Anwendung von Tierarzneimitteln, Tierseuchenbekämpfung, Tierkörperbeseitigung, Vermeidung von Immissionen sowie Weidetierhaltung. Alle Anforderungen zu diesen Unterkapiteln sind in folgenden Gesetzen geregelt: Tierschutzgesetz, Futtermittelgesetz, Arzneimittelgesetz, Tierseuchengesetz, Tierkörperbeseitigungsgesetz und Immissionsschutzrecht.

Für den Fachmann der Tierernährung ist es interessant, daß nach Anlage 3 zur Futtermittelverordnung zum Zeitpunkt der Erarbeitung des Buches (das Manuskript wurde am 10. Januar 1986 abgeschlossen) elf Gruppen von zugelassenen Zusatzstoffen existierten und zwar folgende: Antioxidantien, Aromastoffe, Zusatzstoffe zur Verhütung bestimmter Tierkrankheiten, die verbreitet auftreten, Emulgatoren, Stabilisatoren, Verdickungs- und Siliermittel, färbende Stoffe, Fließ- und Preßhilfsmittel, Gerinnungshilfsstoffe, Konservierungsstoffe, Verbindungen von Spurenelementen, Vitamine und Provitamine. Die Zulassung von bestimmten Zusatzstoffen ist mit Bestimmungen verbunden, z. B. an welche Tierart der Zusatzstoff in Mischfuttermitteln verfüttert werden darf, bis zu welchem Höchstalter der Tiere die Verfütterung zulässig ist, wie lange die Wartezeit zwischen letzter Fütterung und Schlachtung ist, welche Mindest- und Höchstgehalte an Zusatzstoffen in den Futtermitteln einzuhalten sind, welche Abgabebeschränkungen bestehen.

Bestimmte Zusatzstoffe, welche die Futterverwertung verbessern, bzw. zur Verhütung bestimmter Tierkrankheiten dienen, Carotinoide, Verbindungen von Spurenelementen, Vitamine und Provitamine, sind in Vertrieb und Verarbeitung eingeschränkt. Diese Zusatzstoffe dürfen ausschließlich an Betriebe abgegeben werden, die gewerbsmäßig Vormischungen herstellen. Die Vormischbetriebe dürfen die unter Verwendung dieser Zusatzstoffe hergestellten Vormischungen nur an anerkannte Hersteller von Mischfuttermitteln abgeben. Die Anerkennung als Hersteller von Mischfuttermitteln erfolgt durch die nach Landesrecht zuständige Behörde. Wer diese Zusatzstoffe oder Vormischungen in den Verkehr bringt, ist für die Einhaltung der Abgabevorschriften verantwortlich.

Interessant ist auch, daß der Weidegang der Tiere eine Fütterung im Sinne des Futtermittelrechts darstellt. So z. B. ist in der Anlage 5 zur Futtermittelverordnung für Grünfutter einschließlich Weidegras und Rübenblätter, Grünfuttersilage sowie Heu der Höchstgehalt an Blei auf 40 mg/kg festgesetzt (bei 88 % TS-Gehalt gerechnet). Jedoch darf der Landwirt im eigenen Betrieb erzeugtes Grünfutter bis zu einem Höchstgehalt von 100 mg Blei/kg verfüttern, dabei muß er durch eine entsprechende Beifütterung dafür sorgen, daß er z. B. beim Mastrind 30 mg Blei/kg oder bei Milchrindern 40 mg/kg in der Gesamtration nicht überschreitet. Grünfutter mit mehr als 100 mg Blei/kg darf der Landwirt überhaupt nicht verschneiden und nicht verfüttern.

Diese wenigen interessanten Beispiele sollen die Exaktheit der Darstellung gesetzlicher Bestimmungen – jedoch auch die Verständlichkeit des Textes schwieriger juristischer Verfügungen – darlegen.

Das Buch enthält einleitend ein Abkürzungsverzeichnis, ein Gesetzesverzeichnis und das Literaturverzeichnis.

Ein ausführliches Sachregister erleichtert abschließend die Orientierung in dem umfangreichen Gesamtwerk.

Insgesamt dürfte das vorliegende Buch nicht nur für Fachleute in der BRD von Interesse sein, sondern zur vergleichenden Analyse auch in anderen Ländern gerne studiert werden.

H. Bergner

Melken, Milch vom Euter zum Tank. Verfasser: Alfons Gottschalk. Erschienen im Verlag Eugen Ulmer, Stuttgart, 2. durchgesehene Auflage, 1986; 119 Seiten mit 90 Abbildungen und 22 Tabellen, kartoniert, Format 17×22,5 cm; Preis: DM 19,80

Das vorliegende Buch ist in der Reihe *Tierzuchtbücherei* (Herausgeber Prof. Dr. Horst Kräusslich, München) erschienen. Der Herausgeber Dr. Alfons Gottschalk ist Mitarbeiter in der Bayerischen Landesanstalt für Tierzucht, Grub. Weitere Autoren dieses Buches sind: Ewald Rosenberger (Tierzuchtamt Miesbach), Andreas Mager (Bayerische Landesanstalt für Tierzucht, Grub), Wilhelm Kummer (Staatliche Lehr- und Versuchsanstalt, Almesbach).

Das Buch untergliedert sich in folgende Kapitel: Milch, Milchbildung und Milchgewinnung, Aufbau einer Melkanlage, Melkanlagen, Zusatzgeräte und -einrichtungen, Melken mit der Maschine, Reinigung und Desinfektion der Melkanlage, Wartung und Pflege der Melkanlage, Milchbehandlung im Erzeugerbetrieb, Milchqualität und Milchbezahlung, Züchtung auf Euterqualität sowie Melkberatung und Melkausbildung.

Die Hälfte des Buches ist der Melktechnik und der Milchbehandlung im Erzeugerbetrieb gewidmet. Hierbei wird vom Handmelken bis zu den verschiedenen Melkanlagen (8 verschiedene Systeme sind aufgeführt) umfangreiche Information und Anleitung geboten. Auch die Milchkühlung mit Wärmerückgewinnung im geschlossenen System bzw. offenen System wird beschrieben und der energetische Nutzen belegt. So werden pro Kuh und Jahr bei einer Milchleistung von 4744 kg für Milchkühlung und Warmwasserbereitung 115 kWh im Falle der Wärmerückgewinnung benötigt, dagegen wurden alleine für die Warmwasserbereitung mittels Elektroboiler 345 kWh benötigt und somit liegt der Gewinn pro Kuh und Jahr bei 230 kWh.

Im Rahmen des neuen Bewertungsschemas für die Keimzahl (ab 1. 1. 1986 in der BRD gültig) wird für die Bewertungsstufe 1 die Keimzahl von 500000 auf 300000 herabgesetzt, für die Stufe 2 von 2,5 Mill. auf 1 Mill., für die Stufe 3 von 4 Mill. auf 3 Mill. und die Stufe 4 = oberhalb der genannten Werte der Stufe 3 (Zahlen je cm^3).

Das Unterkapitel im Rahmen der Milchqualität „*Qualitätsbezahlung*" ist für die BRD gültig und interessant hinsichtlich der Bezahlung nach Fettgehalt und Eiweißgehalt sowie den Zu- und Abschlägen für Güteklasse, Zellzahl und Hemmstoffe.

Alle Kapitel werden durch Merksätze untermauert, die auch im Druck farblich sehr gut betont werden. Ein Sachregister beschließt das Buch.

Innerhalb von 4 Jahren konnte die 2. Auflage erscheinen, und auch sie wird bei Auszubildenden und Praktikern wieder großen Anklang finden.

H. Bergner

INHALT

СОДЕРЖАНИЕ

ARCHIVES OF ANIMAL NUTRITION
ARCHIV FÜR TIERERNÄHRUNG

VOLUME 37 JUNE 1987 NUMBER 6

CONTENTS

Archives of Animal Nutrition is indexed in Current Contents/Agriculture, Biology & Environmental Sciences, and abstracted in Nutrition Abstracts & Reviews and in Chemical Abstracts.

FSC
www.fsc.org
MIX
Papier | Fördert
gute Waldnutzung
FSC® C083411

Zeitfracht Medien GmbH
Ferdinand-Jühlke-Straße 7
99095 Erfurt, Deutschland
produktsicherheit@kolibri360.de